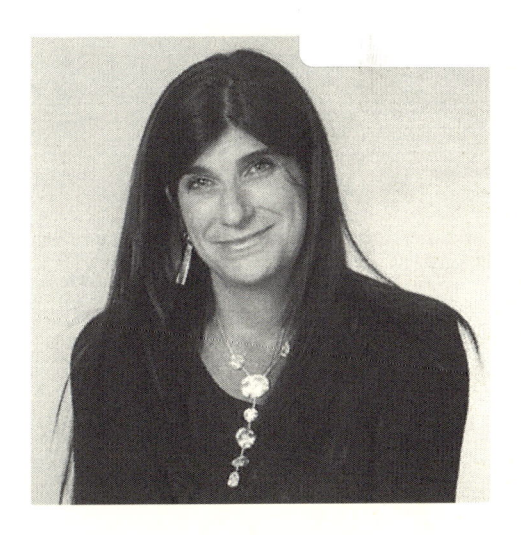

Joanne Fedler's books have been published in the UK, Australia, Germany, Czechoslovakia, Croatia and South Africa. In 2008, *Weiberabend (Secret Mothers' Business)* was on *Der Spiegel*'s bestseller list and has sold more than 150,000 copies worldwide. Joanne studied law at Yale and is a former women's rights advocate, counsellor of abused women, and CEO of a not-for-profit advocacy centre. She writes for *Vogue*, teaches life-writing classes and is a motivational speaker. Joanne has done work to raise money for abused women, breast cancer research and post-natal depression. She lives in Sydney with her husband and two children. You can visit her website at www.joannefedler.com.

Other titles by this author
The Dreamcloth (Jacana Media, 2005)
Secret Mothers' Business (Allen & Unwin, 2006)
Things Without a Name (Allen & Unwin, 2008)

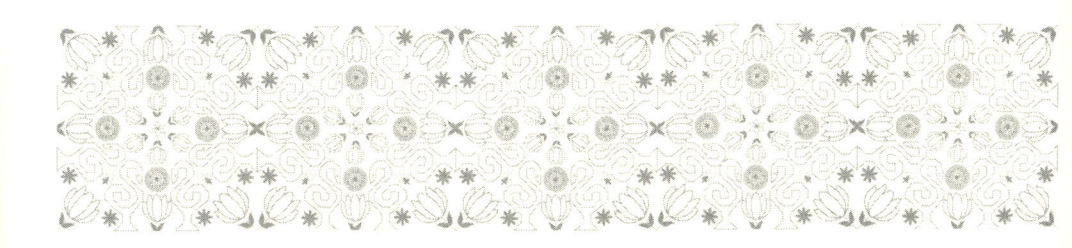

WHEN HUNGRY, EAT

Joanne Fedler

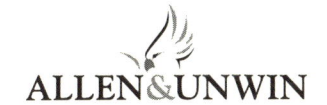

ALLEN&UNWIN

First published in 2010

Copyright © Joanne Fedler 2010

All rights reserved. No part of this book may be reproduced or transmitted in any form or by any means, electronic or mechanical, including photocopying, recording or by any information storage and retrieval system, without prior permission in writing from the publisher. The Australian *Copyright Act 1968* (the Act) allows a maximum of one chapter or 10 per cent of this book, whichever is the greater, to be photocopied by any educational institution for its educational purposes provided that the educational institution (or body that administers it) has given a remuneration notice to Copyright Agency Limited (CAL) under the Act.

Allen & Unwin
83 Alexander Street
Crows Nest NSW 2065
Australia
Phone: (61 2) 8425 0100
Fax: (61 2) 9906 2218
Email: info@allenandunwin.com
Web: www.allenandunwin.com

Cataloguing-in-Publication details are available
from the National Library of Australia
www.librariesaustralia.nla.gov.au

ISBN 978 1 74175 573 2

Set in 12/16 pt Bembo by Bookhouse, Sydney
Printed and bound in Australia by Griffin Press

10 9 8 7 6 5 4 3

Mixed Sources
Product group from well-managed
forests, and other controlled sources
www.fsc.org Cert no. SGS-COC-005088
© 1996 Forest Stewardship Council

Contents

Author's note or *Why you should read this book even if you're skinny*   xi

PART ONE   *Hunger*

  1   The food fascist   3
  2   Bottoming out   10
  3   Seconds   17
  4   Leftovers   23
  5   Shortbread   28
  6   *Schmaltz*   34
  7   Grub   40
  8   Shiver   45
  9   Reap   53
10   Greenhorns   58
11   Rage   65
12   Convert   71
13   Scoff   75
14   Laurels   81

PART TWO   *Hope*

15   Cracks   87
16   Banana   92
17   Blue sky   98
18   Small bites   104
19   Coincidence #1   108
20   Run   113
21   Consumption   119

22	Crisp	*124*
23	A ghastly poetry	*129*
24	Burp	*133*
25	Coincidence #2	*138*
26	God	*143*
27	Boss	*151*

PART THREE *Heartbreak*

28	The list	*157*
29	10,000 steps	*164*
30	Panic	*168*
31	Mash	*174*
32	The sign	*178*
33	*Tzimtzum*	*183*
34	Seven	*186*
35	Fork	*191*
36	Plate	*195*
37	A full table	*198*
38	Forever	*204*
39	Rock	*208*
40	Curb	*213*
41	Shaken	*217*
42	Going	*220*
43	Comrades	*226*

PART FOUR *Humility*

44	Arriving hungry	*231*
45	Empty	*239*
46	Outside	*243*
47	Fat cat	*251*
48	Extra virgin	*254*

49	Zilch	*264*
50	Small fry	*267*
51	Snap	*276*
52	Seed	*279*
53	Rite	*284*
54	Eyeball	*291*
55	Rearview	*294*
56	Chop wood	*298*
57	Training	*307*

PART FIVE *Home*

58	Return	*313*
59	Roots	*318*
60	Sweet and sour	*322*
61	Coincidence #3	*325*
62	Angels	*332*
63	Swim	*338*
64	Digest	*343*

Epilogue	*349*
Appendix: *An eating meditation, or spiritual principals, for losing weight, leaving home or letting go*	*351*
Stuff I read while I was hungry	*354*
Glossary	*359*
Acknowledgements	*367*

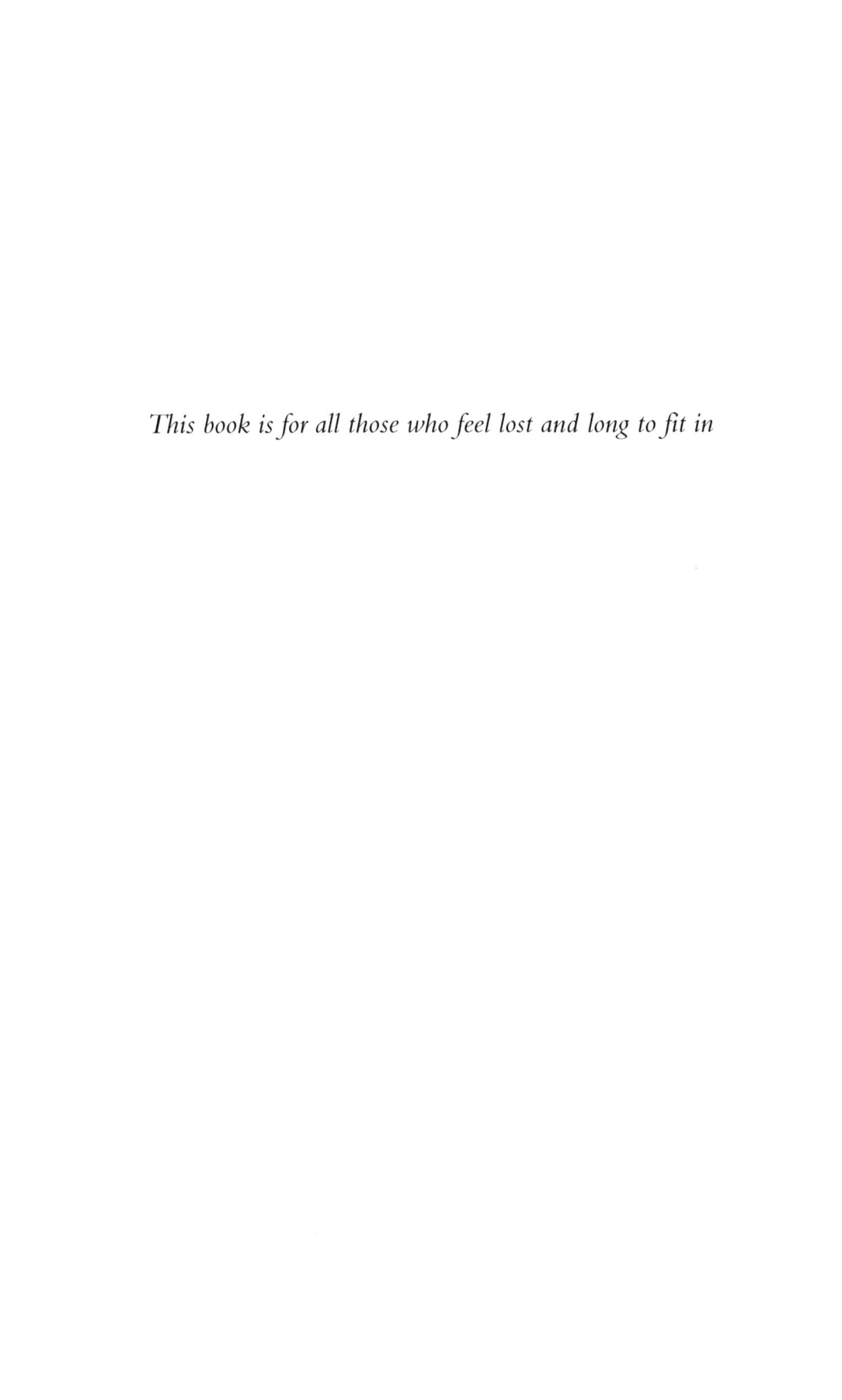

This book is for all those who feel lost and long to fit in

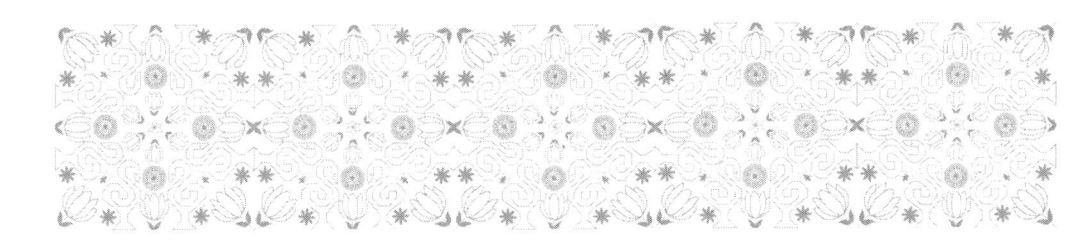

Author's note
or Why you should read this book even if you're skinny

Autobiography is the verbal equivalent of streaking, and at my age there should probably be a law against that. What streakers fail to appreciate is that not everyone wants a close encounter with their uglies. Some people get astonishingly offended by nudity, especially if there's a bit of blubber involved. Unfortunately, a degree of exhibitionism is unavoidable when you write about your own life, an impulse perhaps most generously understood as the garrulous need to share one's neuroses with as large an audience as possible.

I love a good voyeuristic peek into other peoples' lives just as much as the next person. Through the memoirs of mountain climbers and anthropologists who've lived with monkeys I've picked up all sorts of useful parenting skills, even though I can assure you I've no intention of climbing Mount Kilimanjaro nor of taking up residence with creatures who de-lice one another to pass the time. What I've come to understand is that there are only so many steps in this human dance. The diverse details of a life don't divide us as much as the common insights unite us, which is why this story about a mother leaving her homeland and losing weight might interest you, even if you've never done either, or if motherhood is not your destiny for any reason, including a set of testicles.

By the time my fortieth birthday loomed, I'd married, had two kids, left the country of my birth for another and picked up plenty of baggage along the path. I was long overdue for a spiritual spring-clean. But I couldn't very well take a year off to meditate in an ashram. Who was going to make the lunch boxes?

So instead, I opted for doing something about the fatty deposits on my rear end before they fossilised.

And that's where this story begins. Or so I thought.

I started a new eating plan of smaller portions and more mindful eating hoping to get thinner. But as my relationship with food began to slowly change, and the weight peeled off me, gram by obstinate gram, I was brought to a place of much 'greater hunger', as Laurens van der Post calls it, which had nothing to do with what I put in my mouth. What began as a mission to get back into a bikini became a pilgrimage towards acceptance, which was neither on my food list nor my itinerary.

To lose weight, give up a bad habit or leave something or someone behind, we're forced to let go. When we start over we have to metabolise our loss and fit in again. I don't think it matters whether it's a foreign culture, a new way of being, or size 10 pants.

A measure of hyperbole and caricature are to be expected when people sculpt their own stories. Though I have, to the best of my ability, been true and open about my own emotions,

AUTHOR'S NOTE

I owe the innocent people who are inadvertently major players in my life some privacy and respect. Consequently, some of the names in this book have been changed, and direct attributions camouflaged, to ensure these people will continue to talk to me. To each of them I extend my greatest love, thanks and respect for being part of the abundant feast of my life.

Joanne Fedler, Sydney 2010

Part One

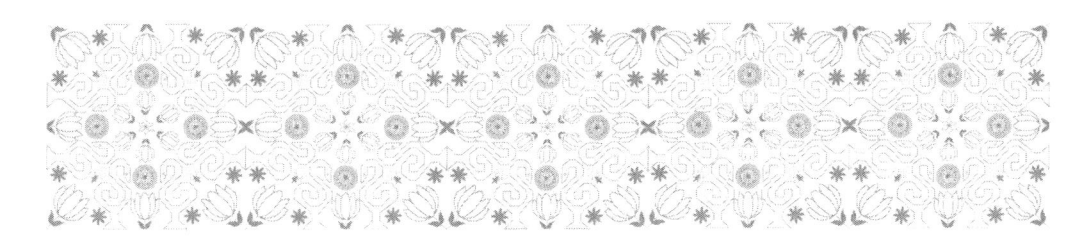

Hunger

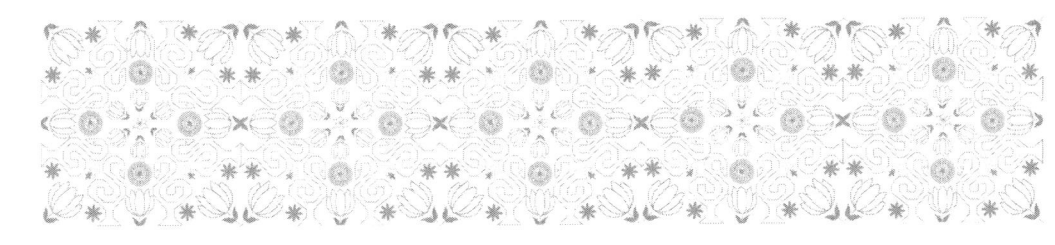

1
The food fascist

Hunger pushes the hippopotamus out of the water.
LUO PROVERB

I wish I'd never kept this appointment.

But regret has come too late. I've just received some very bad news from a stick insect in a miniskirt: I am 'obese'. Yes, that is the word she has chosen from an extensive treasury of adjectives to describe someone who is carrying a bit of extra weight, principally around the thighs, belly and buttocks. 'Obese' is, I'm hoping, dietician-speak for 'You could lose a few kilos'.

She's holding a kilojoule-counting book and a food diary in which, if I am *Serious About Losing Weight*, I must record every morsel that passes my lips, as if I were tagging evidence for a murder trial.

Apparently this is *The Only Way*. 'Do you or do you not want to lose weight?' she asks. She's not interested in any excuses. She's heard them all. Her approach may be harsh but it's effective. She's not here to be my friend. I'm so glad she's cleared that up.

To add to the indignity, I am to wear a pedometer and do 10,000 steps a day. Not one less. To boost my 'sluggish metabolism'. I detest words like 'sluggish', which bring to mind mollusc-like inertia, and make a person feel akin to those flabby bits one is awfully keen to get rid of.

Until this moment I've never had a problem with the word 'obese'. I never minded it when it didn't apply to me.

She must be exaggerating – this scrawny, officious creature – for effect; to shock. As if her exorbitant fee wasn't brutal enough. Apparently only when you pay for something, and it hurts, do you appreciate its value. Somewhere in there she throws in the terminology of self-worth.

I glance down at my blubbery belly across which my hands are folded. My Granny Bee taught me to 'never say anything unless you have something nice to say'. I manage to restrain myself from unevolved retorts illustrating my previous desirability: that incident in the women's cloakroom; on the bonnet of my car in the moonlight. I've had men lose their sensibilities and propriety, you know. I've been sexy. I have.

It wasn't so long ago that I'd have worked myself up into a feminist frenzy and verbally guillotined anyone for making a woman feel less human because of her shape or size. I'm a big fan of *The Beauty Myth*, though it's not lost on me that its author, Naomi Wolf, is a luscious size 10 or thereabouts. Ugliness is entirely tolerable when it's not our personal affliction.

But things have changed. *I* have changed. I can barely remember the warrior I once was. I left her behind four years ago, along with everything else I understood about myself when Zed and I made the soul-splicing decision to take our two children away from the intensifying violence in South Africa and bring them to another land boasting dangers of

THE FOOD FASCIST

a different sort, including the most poisonous spiders, snakes and jellyfish known to humankind.

Now here I am, sitting in plush rooms on the lower North Shore of Sydney, Australia, a universe away from my homeland, looking a Food Fascist in the eye.

'I've found it hard, since we left South Africa,' I whimper. She looks back at me, bored. She spends all day castigating large people for their flab with those pursed lips. The world is full of fatties. Obesity is a huge problem in Australia. I'm not alone. But right now, I feel it. Absolutely, utterly alone.

'Is that the excuse you're going to use the rest of your life? "I'm fat because I immigrated"?' she sort of sniggers. 'I've heard them all. Do you have any other excuses, while we're at it?'

I look down at my hands. As if she's so perfect with her neat office, the photo of her smiling family on her desk – all those skinny, pretty teenage girls who eat right and exercise enough – and those lumps of plastic lard labelled 1kg, 5kg, 10kg to 'give people a real sense of how revolting it is to carry this around on your body'.

'I also used to be fat,' she says. 'And I was miserable. Believe me, *nothing tastes as good as thin feels.*'

The Food Fascist fat? There *is* the intense rigour of the convert about her. I begin to feel a little light-headed. I can't remember when last I ate. Impending deprivation. My family and I have had to absorb so much loss, relocating to this expensive, cut-throat city halfway across the world. I want to go now, but she's not done. There is more, much more to come.

She tells me to 'stop thinking about food' and to 'take control over my eating habits', as if they're toddlers going through the tantrum phase. But that's so easy to say and so hard to do.

Being overweight is a humiliation all of its own. It comes replete with an entire culture of emotions – shame, guilt, fear, powerlessness. In the past few years, every word I've ever used to describe myself has been snatched away. Back in South Africa, I was considered successful, competent, an expert. In those days when I ran my own organisation and debated politicians on national television, I could never have imagined that one photograph on the beach on Jordan's fifth birthday could make me feel such a sunken human failure. I knew I was a size 18 pants or thereabouts. But pants' size is just a number; those rolls of flab were a geographical phenomenon. The double chin. Like anyone needs two. I looked at that photograph and I said aloud, 'That is not me,' as if someone else was wearing my blue bathing suit and lighting my child's birthday candles. And I swear, I have never, until that moment, indulged in enough vanity to actually tear up a photograph of myself. But I did tear that photo up. Into tiny bits.

But then, if it wasn't me, who was it? Someone I'd become, inadvertently, incrementally, through the haze of early motherhood and immigration. While the real me wasn't paying attention and was feeling sorry for her pathetic, exiled self, shorn of her achievements and dreams in a life given up.

There's no way I can share these intimacies with the Food Fascist. For one thing, she clearly doesn't give a shit. And my time is almost up. There's a room of other obese people out there waiting to pay her for her sneer.

I'm close to tears but I don't want to cry in front of her. An obese person in tears is just that much more pathetic than a dry-eyed fatso. Admittedly, I've come here of my own volition. I really do want to be reunited with my cheekbones, my collarbones, my hipbones (the long-lost relatives of my youth), which all got swallowed in the quicksand of my pregnancies. I don't want to be fat and forty.

THE FOOD FASCIST

But I don't want to be told that I'm obese or, for that matter, anything other than just lovely and brave for having made this appointment. I know I'm twenty-four kilos heavier than I was before I had kids, when 'slim' could sit alongside my name without needing a special visa. I realise it shouldn't have come to the point where I needed to pay someone else to a) tell me what I already knew, and b) abuse me for not working it out all by myself.

I understand that until we stop making the same mistakes, the universe will keep giving us opportunities to learn the lessons we need, like a pop-up you just can't click away. But right now I'm not thinking any of this. I'm thinking the Food Fascist is probably sexually repressed which is why she's such a bitch.

I wonder if there's a medical condition I can blame. Regrettably, I don't have a metabolism problem. My thyroid is in tip-top shape. I'm not a chocoholic nor a secret eater. I eat mostly salads, fresh fruit juices, sushi and stir-fries. Lots and lots and lots of them. And so, each year, a few kilos have snuck in and, because I'm tall, it's hardly showed. Until now.

The problem is: I love food. It's not some neurotic eating disorder I inherited from my teens, nor do I have self-image issues. Zed loves me, and has never found me – even at my heaviest – less than ridiculously desirable (God bless him). I just love food. I read recipe books the way some people read Stephen King. Salivating is one of my hobbies. *What am I going to cook tonight?* is possibly my favourite thought. How people feed you is the measure of how they love you.

People who love you never say 'You've had enough'. They always say 'Have some more'. More is love. Less is rejection.

The Food Fascist breaks my reverie: 'Don't think of this as a diet, think of it as an eating plan,' she says.

'But it *is* a diet,' I whimper.

'Don't use that word – it's banned from your vocabulary.'

I've got to watch what comes out of my mouth as well as what goes in? This is surely too much to bear.

'I want you to be hungry,' the calorie-counting whippet says to me.

Hungry? Other than it being a word I associate with World Vision, I can't say when last I felt that sensation.

'But I love food,' I tell her. I detect a small whine in my voice.

'Love it a little less,' she says strictly.

Sitting across from her, I feel a vaguely familiar sensation. I'm being dumped. The tears return to my eyes and this time I can't staunch the flow. All the loss I've experienced over the last few years rolls down my cheeks. I hate goodbyes. I've said too many of those. Being hungry means saying goodbye all over again to my friends: olive bread, green curry, Ferrero Rocher chocolates, Cabernet Sauvignon…

As I hand over her fee of $160, which is a week's worth of groceries, for the half-hour I've spent in a state of part-humiliation, part-justification, I realise I just wanted someone to be nice to me. To tell me I wasn't really fat. That everything will be alright. That we made the right decision uprooting our little family and coming to Australia. That a few extra kilos are actually perfectly okay, and will be easy to get rid of. Like my homesickness. My culture shock. My heartache.

None of these consolations is forthcoming. She hands me a receipt. 'You can claim some of it back from your private healthcare fund.'

I fold the receipt and put it in my bag. The little pedometer clicks away. I'm afraid. Of being hungry. Of letting go. Of losing things.

'Make friends with hunger,' she tells me, with a little humanity in her voice as she shoos me out her office.

Later, I'll come to understand that everything I hate, everything that's causing me pain and anger is, in my adored Sufi poet Rumi's words, 'where the light enters'.

Without knowing it, the Food Fascist is delivering me a profound message that I'm unable, in this moment of self-pity, to hear. Over the next months and years it will sink in, first to my growling empty belly, and later to parts of me that are yearning to have a much deeper hunger filled.

Hunger, it's going to turn out, will be one of my kindest teachers. And the Food Fascist, an angel. Albeit in a fabulous disguise.

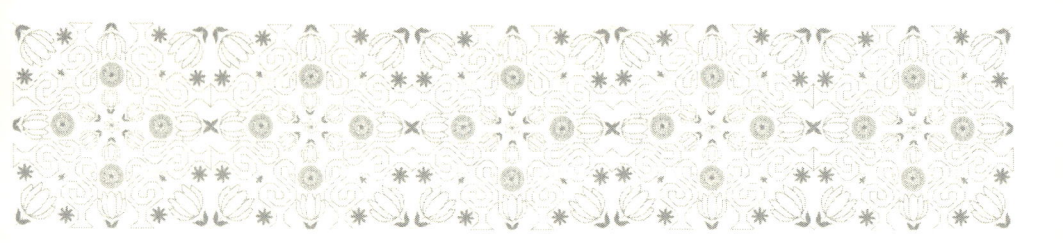

2
Bottoming out

It isn't done as easily as it is said.
YIDDISH PROVERB

Okay, so this is probably a good time to let you know that this isn't a book about how to lose weight. I've got nothing against How-To books as a rule, but this isn't one of them. I'm also not going to bore you with the details of my daily kilojoule intake, nor the litres of water I drank, urinated out or retained. That's what personal trainers are for.

But this is a story of loss in the 'how-it-ties-into-the-big-picture-of-life's-meaning' kind of way, which I was amazed to discover has some unexpected overlaps with calories.

See, as a diligent Virgo Type-A personality, I'd been working towards the spiritual imperatives of health, wealth and happiness for ages. To fail at any of them felt like a concession of stupidity or illiteracy, or a tragic combination of both. I'd read enough self-help literature in my life to know that the basics of living a healthy, happy life are neither rocket science nor a secret. We have to eat less, exercise more and avoid fatty foods to lose weight. We have to forgive, own our own shit, be generous and grateful to be happy. We all know this, right? But there's always been this gap – a Bermuda Triangle – between what I knew intellectually and what I did in my daily life. My battle, which I suspect is maybe the human battle, has always been to translate what I 'know' into who I am.

It didn't seem to matter how fast I could read the next Five-Steps-To-Emotional-Health or Power-of-Awakening, the tortoise of the heart moves at its own speed. The space between the talk and the walk is probably a microscopic distance of synapses, but it's equally a mysterious conversation between the mind, the soul and the quadriceps, and it's *this* exchange that intrigues me.

Dotted around my house are statues of dozens of little Buddhas I've collected over the years, eyes closed with a mesmerising smile on their lips. I love these little statues because a) they make me feel a whole lot better about the size of my belly, and b) that smile comes from a place I long to reach of equal non-attachment to suffering or to pleasure, a place where I just *know* that mysterious conversation between the mind, the soul and the body is happening.

Legend has it that Siddhartha Gautama, more commonly known as the Buddha, spent many days and nights in contemplation under the Bodhi tree. When he finally stood up to stretch his legs in a state of enlightenment, he claimed meditation was one of the paths to eternal bliss, though it's obvious Buddha wasn't the primary carer of small children. Still, I reckon an insight accrued over such a long time without talking is worth a try. So, over the years, I've sat and listened to my breath with the hope of getting a bit of that nirvana-action. And the Buddha wasn't bullshitting – sometimes tiny cracks of space between our thoughts open up, gasps of pure consciousness which soothe the soul, stripping away the gunk of grief, longing, mother-guilt, lust, regret, self-importance, hunger or, indeed, self-loathing over a flabby tummy. Mine generally don't last very long before someone calls me to make two-minute noodles, wipe up cat vomit or dispose of a cockroach carcass. Mystical practice tells us that this awareness of formlessness is who we *really* are, not the shapes, wrinkles and blemishes we see in the mirror, which, speaking for myself, comes as something of a relief.

When I'm able to reach those golden glades of consciousness, I do feel free from the tangle of anguishes in my life, which Buddha expressed as coming from wanting things to be different from what they are. In those moments I'm released from longing, grasping and hoping for more or other things. I am, I guess, happy.

It's a bit of a bugger that this state seems contrary to the hard-wiring of the human personality, which is a natural worrier, dreamer and wuss, scared of loss – especially the biggie, Death. But like it or not, loss can't be avoided. It is, to use the terminology of parenting manuals, a 'compulsory activity' (like bedtime, homework or teeth-brushing). Sometimes in life we choose loss, and sometimes it chooses us. Either way, it's a misery-packed enterprise. I've seen people lose their minds, wallets and innocence and they're all terrifically depressing affairs. To give up anything – smoking, gambling or a rotten marriage – is a gut-wrench, even when the habit is slowly stealing our antioxidants, liver or self-esteem.

I personally don't have an impressive track record in dealing with loss. I simply fall apart, easily and noisily, just as I always scream in movies when the guy jumps out from behind the door. I never get used to the shock, even when I know it's coming (no matter if Zed warns, 'Get ready for a door-jumper').

BOTTOMING OUT

But, with my fortieth birthday looming, the time had come for a bit of adult poise, to renounce my status as a fragile human Jenga tower and to be more like ... like the Eiffel Tower in a thunderstorm: serene, graceful and sturdy. Just like I've advised my kids when dealing with playground bullies to stop playing the role of the victim and to assert their own power, I wondered if I could do the same when loss stole *my* lunch and called *me* names. Because in life, even when we can't choose *whether* we want something to happen, we can still choose *how* to do it or at the very least decide how to *feel* about it.

Could I confront loss as an opportunity to develop some spiritual biceps? A teacher of the truth of the impermanence of all things? A friend who points out what I'm not seeing or avoiding in myself?

And that's where the Food Fascist comes in.

By the time I fronted up to her, two healthy pregnancies had chewed me up and spat me out. My body was like a wetsuit they'd let just one too many fat guys squeeze their lardy arses into. My breasts had exhaled one day and never inhaled again. Gravity is never explained as a form of corporeal cruelty, but it is. Oh it very much is.

I loved and couldn't stand my body in equal parts. My older sister, Carolyn, was born hard-of-hearing so I've always been grateful for having a healthy body with all my senses intact. But in my small-minded, day-to-day dealings with it, I bitched at it for not being healthy *and* thin. Lots of skinny people are flushed with wellbeing and go on to lead long and glamorous lives and I saw no reason why I couldn't be one of them.

Over ten years, I'd successfully raised two fit and healthy children as well as my own weight by twenty-four kilos. Shannon and Jordan had busy exercise routines of swimming, tennis and karate lessons while I sat on the sidelines sipping cappuccinos and eating lunch-box leftovers. Look, I'm not stupid – I knew I needed to exercise but seriously, who's got time? There are days when I didn't get to *wee* when I wanted.

I also felt guilty about the cost of a dietician which would gouge a huge chunk out of our monthly budget when there were Club Penguin memberships, DS Pokemon games, saxophone lessons and the latest Bratz doll competing for priority. Since we'd deprived our kids of everything that was rightfully theirs, including grandparents and cousins, annual holidays and the financial security we'd had in South Africa, I verily *deserved* the short straw.

But, okay. Let's be honest. Excuses aside, the plain fact was that I'd given up. I believed I *couldn't* lose weight. Maybe that was easier than actually doing something about it. For starters, I've always been a 'big' girl. My father had put it to me straight very early on. 'You'll never be a model, my darling,' he'd said when I was fifteen, 'you just aren't built that way,' referring to my 'big bones' and my big nose. 'But,' my dad said, kissing my forehead, 'you will be *other* things.'

Other things?

During my teens, my personal aspirations did not extend beyond the desire for Samuel Finkelstein to French-kiss me. Which by the way, he never did. My parents did their best with what they had, nudging their fat-bottomed girl through adolescence with accolades of how 'striking' and 'special' I was, but they just didn't understand. Samuel Finkelstein liked skinny.

But much as I have, at times in my life, been fit and strong and lithe and supple, I have never ever, not once, even for a brief time, been skinny.

Secondly, over the years I'd put myself through many a diet (Atkins, cabbage soup, lemon detox – the list does go on) and had failed each time. Oh sure, I'd lost a few kilos here and there and often quickly. But it took a while before I got it: speed is a skinny red herring. The quicker it falls off, the quicker it comes back, often with interest. To get permanently rid of every kilo, I needed to learn to do it sloooow, like a deep yogic breath or a tai chi movement. I knew this. I just didn't like the information. I'm also crabbily impatient.

I'd even attended Weight Watchers' classes for close to a year, bought all the recipe books, read all the literature, mounted those scales, and with agonising self-consciousness participated in all those 'share-your-success' renditions of scrumptious low-fat meals in a room full of other people hoping thinness would bring them happiness and meaning. I lost a sensational four kilos over a period of six months (see, I can do slow). And regained them in the week after I stopped counting points. So where had I gone wrong?

By this stage I was also over New Age theory suggesting overweight people need to examine what they're emotionally 'holding onto'. I've never heard anyone crucify a skinny person for what they're afraid to embrace. Maybe I was just *meant* to be the big girl everyone wants to hug. I mean, there are worse things, right?

But there came a point when I looked at my body in the mirror and the last thing I felt that way about was a three-legged dog Jordan spotted down at the beach. Even self-loathing is less depressing than pity. Fur aside, it would've been hard to tell the difference between my stomach and a shar pei's face. I realised that being a mother no-one was looking out to ensure *I* got my two fruits and five veggies a day. I knew I couldn't get my pre-kid body back – I'm not delusional – but something hopeful inside me roared; maybe it was possible to salvage the bits that were still optimistically hanging on. I rationalised that I'd probably screwed my kids up anyway with all the mistakes I'd already made. Having 'selfish' added to their catalogue of parenting complaints (for unilaterally removing pies and fries from the dinner menu) seemed a small price to pay for a decent pair of thighs.

I was wearing the equivalent of two pregnancies in weight so I generously gave myself two years to lose twenty-four kilos. A kilo a month – how hard could that be? I'd seen people on *The Biggest Loser* drop five kilos in *a week*. Okay, so they have daily four-hour exercise sessions with personal trainers coupled with the incentives of public humiliation and a massive cash prize at the end. My point is that it *is* physically possible.

By the time I rallied myself to action, I was sickened by how little control I had over my life (as if any of us ever do). I feel safest and happiest when I'm in control of things. I'm not huge on surprises unless they involve flowers and champagne. I don't, for example, do well in being asked to be completely spontaneous, as in 'Let's-worry-about-where-we-sleep-when-we-get-there'. I like to know what's coming.

I was thirty-eight years old, all my pants were tight and I was very out of love with my body. I didn't need anyone to explain what *that* meant in spiritual terms.

Maybe I was just hoping to fall in love again.

Because unlike the unforgiving body, the heart is a voracious optimist.

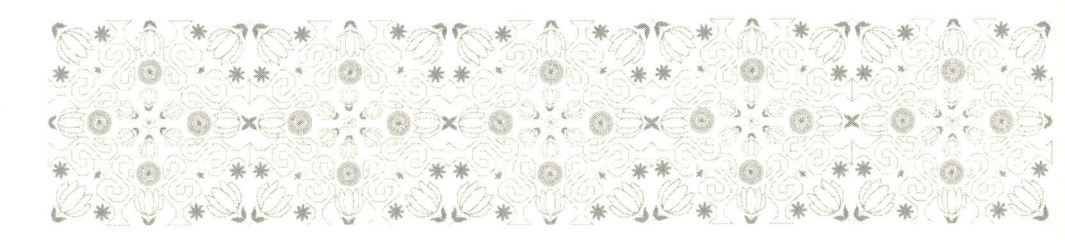

3
Seconds

Strong souls have willpower; weak ones only desires.
CHINESE PROVERB

It's day two of my new 'eating plan' and on my plate is a speck of food I've seen fancy restaurants call *nouvelle cuisine*, which is French for 'no food', and if it isn't it should be. This smidgeon of nutrition is, in fact, my 'dinner'.

The quantity of pasta I'm allowed is – please measure this yourself – half a cup. It works out to exactly fourteen spirals. Okay, so I counted them. It's what I'd normally eat to warm up my eating muscles while dishing up for Zed and the kids. It's what I'd put away while checking if the food needs more salt or another spoon of tomato paste. In the past, a plate of pasta for me was approximately six times this amount. I measure the half cup again, just to be sure. Yep, fourteen. I squash them down a bit to get all the air out – you know how puffy those spirals can be – and manage to squeeze in another three.

I don't care that William Blake saw 'a world in a grain of sand' or that Zed once commented about the wet spot: 'That's a hell of a lot of child support right there.' Feng shui is so full of shit — less is never *more*. This fleck of food is not a feast, not even a metaphoric one. It's just plain small and what I'm struggling with is acceptance. Not to mention that I have to drown out the Jewish mother in me who is right about now having a cadenza.

I toss in a huge handful of rocket and fresh basil leaves plus four stems of steamed asparagus. My modest gathering of spirals is now quite puffed up and seems less pitiful. I grate in some lemon zest and throw in five snow peas. I chop up a birdseye chilli and add that too. I slowly grind black pepper over the foliage of my dinner. There will sadly be no parmesan cheese to join this merrymaking on my plate.

Zed and the kids are seated at the table and start on their pasta hillocks, Zed and Shannon's drenched in bolognaise sauce with an avalanche of parmesan cheese cascading down the side, Jordan's 'just plain'. The aroma of that sauce, maternal love in a blend of tomato, garlic and oregano, makes me salivate.

'Please, don't wait for me, eat up,' I say.

I spear exactly ONE spiral onto my fork with a leaf of rocket. I bite it in half to stretch this meal out, so that I won't be finished long before anyone else. I chew more slowly than probably seems normal for a person with all their own teeth. Between mouthfuls I rest my fork on my plate. I sip my water. I count to ten before picking up my fork again. When I look up, Zed and the kids are staring at me.

Jordan starts to snigger. 'Whachu doing, Mum?' he asks, stuffing a bouquet of spirals into his mouth.

I clear my throat. 'What does it look like? I am Eating My Dinner,' I reply.

'Yours looks Dis. Gus. Ting,' he says chewing open-mouthed.

'Why aren't you having what we're having?' Shannon asks, bolognaise sauce dribbling down her chin.

I hand her a serviette. 'Don't get that on your karate suit – didn't I tell you to take it off before dinner?'

'I didn't hear you,' she says, wiping her cheeks.

'As if,' Jordan says. 'I heard her.'

'Shut up, you weirdo,' Shannon says.

'Can we just be respectful to each other?' I snap.

'Why aren't you having bolognaise?' Shannon repeats.

'I'm trying to lose a little weight,' I say.

'Why, cos you're fat?' Jordan asks.

'I'm . . . slightly . . . overweight, is all,' I say. 'Just a few kilos. And I want to be healthy.'

'Are you sick?' Shannon asks in alarm. Two years ago, her kitten got feline AIDS and had to be put down. Before that, we'd had to give up our cats Rain and Shadow when we left South Africa. Shannon used to love dressing Shadow up with little hoods and other haberdashery. That cat was Buddhistly tolerant of being confused with Strawberry Barbie. Shannon, I'm convinced, carries these losses with her in her tender breast. A few months ago she'd informed me she'd never be able to 'get over' her kitten's death unless we got a replacement, even though we already had a cat, Tanaka. But Tanaka was a cat. Not a kitten. Hence Jinx, the latest addition to our family, who, despite my best efforts, hasn't been able to tell the difference between the cat litter, my favourite fluffy tiger-print Betty Boop slippers and the doonas. Since we've added her to our family, I've been washing bed linen every day and wondering why Shannon had to pick the one kitten from the litter with emotional issues.

'I'm perfectly healthy,' I say reassuringly. 'But I want to be lighter because . . .' – I measure my words, not wanting to dump my anxieties on Shannon who asked me the other day, 'Mum, am I overweight?' when she has a gorgeously perfect nine-year-old build that a boy in her playground saw fit to label 'fat' – '...then I won't put my back out so often. I need to take some heaviness off my spine.'

'And you'll also get pretty and skinny,' she says.

'Your mother is the most beautiful woman in the world,' Zed corrects her.

'To *you*, Dad,' Shannon corrects him.

'Anyway, there are going to be a few changes around here. We are going to be eating more fish. More chicken breast and lots of salads. And I'm not always going to be eating the same things as you.'

'Yuck. I hate fish,' Jordan says. 'And I don't eat salad.'

'Well, you're going to have to learn,' I retort.

'I just won't eat,' he says.

'Fine, be hungry,' I say.

I glance at Zed who quickly takes a slug of his beer. 'I think the Swans are playing the Eagles this weekend,' he says.

'Cool,' Jordan says. 'Aussie Rules.'

I sniff mightily, pick my fork up and aim for an asparagus spear this time.

Zed eats his seconds guiltily. This man can eat as much as he wants. Not only does he have skinny genes, he's also a long-distance runner whose modest ambitions include running a marathon a month and then a marathon in every city of the world. I've stopped trying to understand him. These are alien aspirations of strange people who exercise for fun and get grumpy when they miss a day.

Besides, men burn energy more quickly. They just have to think about losing weight and they drop a pants' size, in much the same way they just think about sex and the body obliges with a triumphant hurrah! A few years ago Zed cut out beer for a month and had to replace his entire wardrobe. I'm not competitive by nature and will happily and defiantly lose at Scrabble, but this is one part of our history I prefer not to discuss.

I have no idea how he and I ended up together – it was a match made in a law-school corridor, through the slow itch of platonic friendship characterised by a lot of teasing which suddenly sprouted into an unexpected romantic rash. Very *When Harry Met Sally*. I feel safe in saying that Zed loves me as I am. Warts and all. A couple of years ago, I had to have a large growth cut out from behind my right knee. It had begun as a little bump but, as the years went by, seemed to be getting bigger and more tender to the touch. It was nothing sinister, but Zed was *sad* when I had it removed. He would always tuck his hand behind my knee in bed and play with it. 'It was a disgusting growth,' I told him.

'Yes, but it was *your* growth,' he said fondly.

You will understand that it is a waste of time for me to explain to Zed my need to lose twenty kilos or so.

It's impossible not to love a man like this to the very frontiers of my affection, which is one reason we're still together after everything we've been through. The other reason is that he really is the least irritating person I know. And I get irritated very easily.

Shannon asks if she can have more. For a moment – and it really is just a moment – I think of that cruel playground jibe and wonder if I should try to distract her with *The Simpsons* or some other non-consumable treat. The Food Fascist made certain I understood that going for seconds is a neurological fault of the brain. It takes fifteen to twenty minutes after eating for the brain to register fullness in the body. Seconds happen in the information hiatus between the head and the belly. Despite this, seconds, especially around my table, is a basic human right. I have known this intuitively since I saw *Oliver* as a child.

'Sure,' I mutter, getting up to dish up another helping of pasta and bolognaise sauce.

I do several large lunges on my way to the kitchen. Lunges, I'll have you know, burn a lot of fat.

4
Leftovers

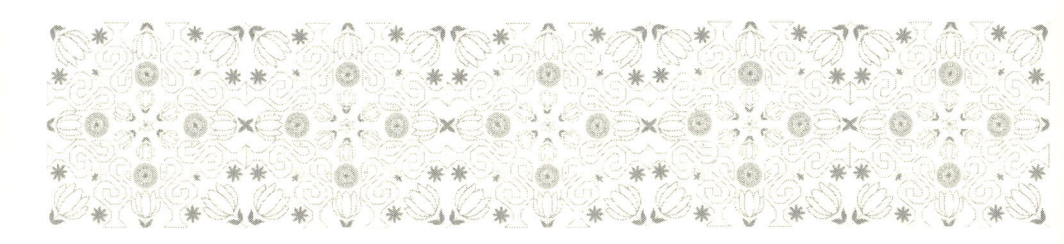

You learn a lot about a man by his behaviour when hungry.

ZAMBIAN PROVERB

I've always looked forward to dinner at the end of a long day of mothering chores, when my family and I can sit down around the table and natter in between mouthfuls of something delicious I've cooked up or picked up. But by day three of my new eating plan, dinner has become a slow ritual of torture. *Comfort* no longer jumps to mind in word association with *food* as a prompt. None of this touchy-feely, huggy-kissy rapport we once had. Food is like a friend turned Scientologist, and we have nothing to say to each other any more.

But hunger has made this clear: the Food Fascist is a sadist. I'm generally a good people-reader, but perhaps on this occasion I was distracted by my *obesity*. How else to explain that she has only allowed me two carbohydrates at dinner? A glass of wine is one carbohydrate. Have you ever considered how cheerless it is to be forced to choose between a roast potato and a glass of Chardonnay? For breakfast I can have a protein *or* a carbohydrate. No egg on toast. What sort of a sick freak makes you pick between the egg and the toast? Before I'd left her rooms, the Food Fascist had looked me in the eye and right into my very soul before saying: 'It's okay to throw food away. I want you to leave food on your plate. Don't just eat because it's there.'

She didn't seem to understand. Over-catering is the involuntary reflex of a Jewish heritage. I always make large enough portions so no-one (including a stranger and his extended family who may perchance pitch up uninvited at our door) will go hungry. But in the past few days, as I'm no longer in the running for seconds, we've been swamped with leftovers. The fridge has become a hodgepodge of Tupperware, unidentifiable tin-foiled shapes and re-sealed tubs that make me anxious. I come from Africa where people are starving, right at this very moment. I could probably even name a few. For this reason I can only bring myself to throw food away when a mould is so set in it could cure a disease.

But I'm in Australia now, a land of plenty, excess and abundance, a planet apart from the harsh realities of South African life, where you can leave empty cartons and old newspapers outside and by morning the homeless will have scavenged them for roofing, bedding, crockery – even art. In Africa, people make their livelihoods from 'rubbish', inventing tin craft, number-plate bags, bottle-top ornamentation or telephone-wire sculpture, things that inspire the human spirit in their reinterpretation of 'junk'. We've been in Australia for four years now and I still wince when I see council trucks churning perfectly good furniture and other household items into scrap. I have to force myself not to think about how many homes in South Africa's townships could be fitted with beds and furniture with the rejects of Sydney's suburbs. In the pouch of that thought all my pain, my loss and my sorrow are tucked. I come from a place which taught me to abhor waste. But this antipathy isn't a good enough reason for something to end up in my mouth. If I don't learn to cook less, leave food on my plate or throw leftovers away, it will go to my waist.

I don't want to have to endure the indignity of my last encounter at Franklins supermarket where the woman behind me in line at the check-out had inquired with idiotic brutality and a large grin, 'So, when are you due?'

Bracing myself I'd said, 'Actually, I've already had my children. These,' prodding my belly, 'are the leftovers.'

Watching her squirm was a pyrrhic victory, for there's only so much joy in witnessing someone's social anguish at a *faux pas* essentially at your expense.

And I decided then and there that I don't want to be wearing leftovers anymore.

'What's that noise?' Zed asks, sitting up in bed.

'It's my stomach,' I hiss.

'Oh . . .' He shrugs. 'Sorry.'

'Yeah, sorry to wake you,' I say. 'Hungry people find it hard to sleep.'

'You've been very . . .' I can see Zed scrambling for the right phrase, one that will not incite me to bop him on the nose, 'disciplined,' he says.

'If you'd met the Food Fascist, you'd be disciplined too,' I tell him. 'She's a scary bitch from hell.'

'Are you doing this for you or her?' he asks.

'She called me "obese",' I say into my pillow.

'You're not,' he says kindly.

'I am,' I say, 'according to her charts ...'

'You can stop this diet anytime. No-one's holding a gun to your head,' he says.

I snivel into my pillow. It's a metaphor that haunts me, not that I've personally ever had a gun held to my head. But the fear of it is what finally brought us to Australia where I am safe, but rather unhappy. Should we have stayed in South Africa, I always wonder, where I was happy but scared? In that beautiful country, connected to its people and all its problems, Zed and I had each grown up under an African sun. We'd laugh at jokes in Afrikaans, a language rich with expressiveness in that guttural way that Yiddish is, both of us almost fluent in it from twelve compulsory school years of studying it. I'd learned Zulu at university and could hold a modest exchange about the weather and my own general wellbeing. Zed and I each had a huge cluster of friendships reaching back to our university days. Why did we give up all that happiness? Oh yes, I remember – it was the fear. Was that real or did I imagine it? And is fear more or less tolerable than loneliness? It's getting my head around these impenetrable koans of immigration that makes it impossible for me to know for sure whether We Did the Right Thing.

That's all I want. Some confirmation deep inside the part of me that is connected to God, and life-on-this-planet-as-a-whole, that we didn't make a huge mistake. But it is silent as the moon tonight. Perhaps it can't get a word in edgewise over the growling of my belly.

Sometimes I wonder if God is just a trick of the heart, a contrivance of the soul to twist what things mean according to its own shape, the way optimists always look on the bright side, or depressives can even castigate sunshine. Tonight I just want God to be as comforting as a double helping of cottage pie on my plate. I want to taste God. And I want to go back for seconds.

'I hate you for taking us out of South Africa,' I say to Zed in a moment of amnesic spitefulness. I know it was a shared decision.

'I'm sorry,' he says, reaching for my hand. 'But, remember, we didn't do it for us... we did it for the kids.'

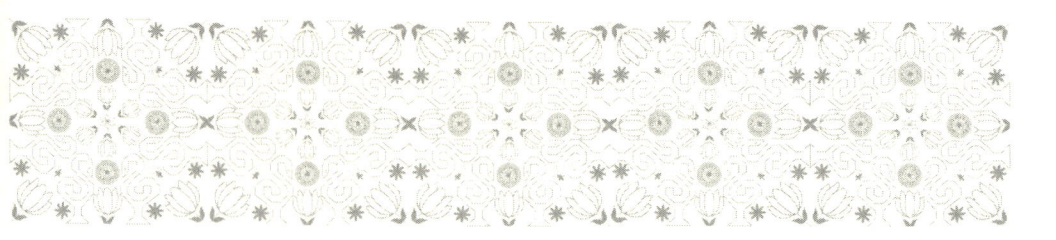

5
Shortbread

Somebody else's body is a faraway nation.
LESOTHO PROVERB

Of course we did it for the kids. I have to keep bringing myself back to that mantra, like returning to the breath in meditation when your mind starts to hitchhike. It's hard to remember who I was before two other people's best interests steered my every decision and waking anxiety. But I was once young and single, if not a little frigid with anger too. To explain I'll take you back some twelve years to a dark little office at the Women's Alliance for Gender Equality (WAGE), a women's crisis centre in Johannesburg, South Africa, where I was working part-time as a legal counsellor. But I'm warning you, it wasn't a happy time.

At WAGE, I learned what real hunger is. I frequently came across people who hadn't eaten proper food in days. They were lethargic and dull-eyed with dry, chapped lips. I saw firsthand what domestic abuse *does* to people, and I'm not talking about the obvious violence. There was the homelessness and the poverty and the emptiness in the faces of women whose spirits had been tortured out of them. There was never a time when I didn't feel both guilty (for not being hungry) and helpless because of the strict client–counsellor boundaries. We weren't allowed to dispense money or food because that would feed dependency and we were supposed to be helping women become independent. I was screamingly hopeless at sticking to the rules, especially when I had cash in my purse or a sandwich in my bag and a starving woman across the desk from me. And I don't use that word 'starving' lightly or hyperbolically, the way one might toss it into a poem about longing, for example.

Australia, despite the language, sunshine and cricket, is very *different* from South Africa. I'm not suggesting there aren't hungry people in Australia (the Food Fascist's clients aside). Poverty sneaks its way into all societies, even one as apparently stable and abundant as Australia, with its robust economy and generous state welfare. But you'd have to be pretty thick not to notice that it takes a particular shine to the third world. The average Australian on a stroll for a morning coffee or newspaper doesn't usually have to step over someone who is, by the World Health Organization's standard, 'at risk of starvation'. But in South Africa, hunger is gracelessly literal.

Every morning at WAGE, one packet of biscuits donated by a large grocery store would be laid out on a paper plate before it was stripped bare by the clusters of women and children, accompanied by cousins, aunts and various in-laws who gathered in WAGE's waiting room in a show of moral support. It was common urban knowledge that at WAGE you could score a free cup of tea with sugar and a shortbread biscuit. Unemployment in South Africa is as unbridled as the violence into which it has inbred, so these women often had nowhere else to go. While my homeland has so much soul, it has problems. Oy, does it have problems.

Violence against women is easily one of its worst, which is why I worked at WAGE as a young, idealistic law graduate instead of at a fancy law firm with espresso machines. Forgetting the idealism which had driven me there in the first place, my work was just plain depressing and repetitive. Stories of abuse are surprisingly unoriginal, the same tale of possessive love, jealousy, drinking, forced sexual contact and cruelty, with minor variations.

I remember Nolwazi, who came in with a broken finger that never got treated and eventually became locked in a crooked curl. When she lifted her blouse to show me her weekend, her torso was patchworked with a tapestry of contusions. The next time I saw her, she had cigarette burns on her arms and tufts of her hair were missing.

'Every time was a comma, this time it's a full stop,' she'd said to me. And this from a woman who'd never been to school or read a book. A psychologist friend of mine who did his doctorate on the use of metaphor in healing once told me that people instinctually use the language of poetry to speak about pain. That made sense to me. Like love, or a pet, I think poetry can help us survive. We secured an AVO against her boyfriend. It didn't really matter how carefully the AVO was worded, because he couldn't read. Literacy is another one of Africa's many insatiable hungers. That AVO was a minor irritation to a man who had a history of stints in jail for petty theft and assault and nothing I could do could fix that.

The cases that shocked me always had a twist – gruesomeness, a fatality, or (God forbid) a child. The few available shelters we begged for spaces had waiting lists that made becoming an organ recipient seem like the twelve-items-or-less queue at Coles. Without this observation taking anything away from my love of small, helpless, furry creatures, there are more shelters for homeless animals in South Africa than there are for abused women.

But Nolwazi was leaving her relationship alive and that was no small victory. A woman can die trying to leave a violent relationship (not infrequently in a manner that rates low down on one's lists of 'preferred ways to die', as death by a hammer to the head or a chisel in the chest tend to).

Mothibi, a young mother with exquisitely braided hair, had a honeyed complexion and the face of an angel – the half that hadn't been permanently disfigured. Her husband had thrown her through a glass window in front of her four-year-old son. She didn't want a divorce or to lay a charge. She wanted an apology. I explained that the law doesn't do 'sorry' and felt like I had to apologise for this failure as if it were my very own fault. All I could offer her was a biscuit and remind her she could come back to us if it happened again. But I never got used to seeing a woman return to the man who'd broken her.

My worst memory, though, is Yvonne. Even though I understand now that she didn't stand a chance, in my dark moments I still go limp with the thought that we failed her. It was just a maintenance court hearing, which is probably why we didn't see it coming. We had an AVO in place, a standard precaution when there were threats of violence. The worst outcome I could have imagined was the magistrate awarding her nothing – I'd seen technicalities work in favour of injustice before, which is why the law can shatter your spirit without even trying. But Yvonne's husband was allowed through security with his firearm because he was a police warden. In court, he pulled it out in full view of a judicial officer and fatally shot her. *To get out of paying maintenance.* He knew he'd be out of the overcrowded cells within the year.

In South Africa, with its history of political prisoners and intermittent release of inmates, the lines between right and wrong often blurred in this way. You learned to develop a certain robustness in the maelstrom of such chaos. Even so, assimilating that level of misogyny is like trying to absorb broken glass through the muscle wall of your heart.

When you hear enough horror stories, the brain performs a fascinating neurological trick. It anaesthetises the natural response of shock, the way flesh will concede a certain numbness if hit too many times, making people pass out into a state of unconsciousness to protect the psyche and the body. Without realising it, this is what was happening to me. It's a form of burnout. But that word doesn't do justice to the incremental withdrawal of emotion from life, a detachment which, over time, fragments the integrity, the inner stitching of the spirit.

Why was I sitting across from women like Nolwazi, listening to horror stories, not being able to help them, and feeling guilty, helpless and, at times, furious and mostly very sad? Good question. My father asked it of me every Friday night when I came for Shabbat dinner.

'God, you look like hell,' he'd say. 'Met any nice abusers lately?'

'I've had a bad week at work,' I'd fume.

'Why on earth do you put yourself through this?' he'd ask. 'It's making you bitter and twisted. Not to mention angry and exhausted.'

Of course my father was right. I was all of those less-than-delightful adjectives. A young woman in her mid-twenties shouldn't be fielding accusations of bitterness, twistedness, anger or exhaustion. It's not an appealing quartet, especially when one is, despite feminist denials to the contrary, eager to get a date with a man with spectacular abdominal muscles.

While working at WAGE, I always felt a hair's-breadth away from uncontrollable fury. Chilled and mellow were hardly the words to describe my response to vaguely sexist remarks about a woman's appearance, life choices or sexual preferences that did not involve her enslaving herself to patriarchy by, say, getting married.

Turning to my father, forgetting for a moment that he was a decent and wonderful man, I'd yell at him: 'Because women are being raped and battered all day, every day, behind closed doors, and because ordinary people like you do nothing, say nothing and just pretend the problem doesn't exist! You've got three daughters, this is also your problem!'

'My darling, have some chicken soup,' my mother would interject.

And, seething, I would.

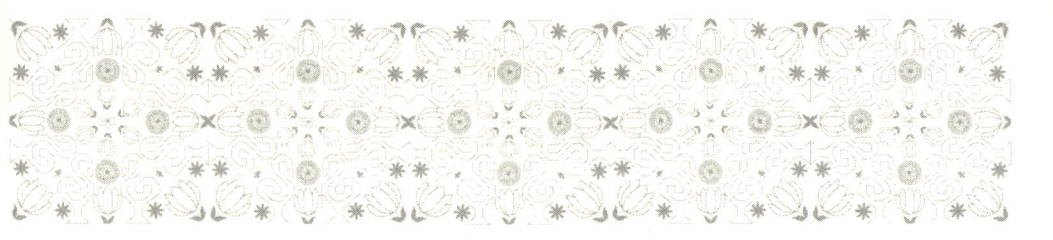

6
Schmaltz

Worries go down better with soup than without.
JEWISH PROVERB

It's been five days since my obesity was brought to my attention and it's hard to think about anything but food. To distract myself, I've made chicken soup. I've done this for two reasons: firstly, chicken soup happens to be one of the six things Jordan will actually eat and secondly, tonight is the Jewish Sabbath and chicken soup, as we all know, is the very soul of Jewish cuisine.

Jewish 'cuisine' is an oxymoron, not being the sort of fare the average person would rush out and pay money for in a restaurant – unless one has a weakness for chopped raw herring, liver, cold beetroot soup, *matza* (flat cardboard-like Passover bread, a ruthless instigator of constipation), *gefilte* fish (fish balls boiled up with fish bones) or sinus-clearing horseradish. Chicken soup proves that while Jews may not find our place amongst the great culinary canons of the world, we do understand the silent love affair between the belly and the heart.

SCHMALTZ

When someone has crippling pneumonia, a particularly drippy head cold or is going through a hideous break-up distended with lawyers, there's really only one thing to do and it doesn't involve overpriced roses or Hallmark sentiments. In such times, love speaks only one language, phrased in ladles of homemade chicken broth.

The making of chicken soup is a gift of biology and genealogy, bundled in there with other specifically Jewish genes like Tay-Sachs disease and keloid scarring. If done right, chicken soup should never taste, as my Granny Bee occasionally remarked with uncharacteristic viciousness about someone's less-than-satisfactory attempt, 'as if the chicken just walked through it'. Chicken soup should be a testament to the very essence of chicken – giblets, claws and all – as if the whole squawking bird had been reduced to golden liquid bones, in an elixir of goodness and marrow and collagen. If properly simmered, it reaches a rich yellow, encouraged by a small sprinkling of turmeric and a bounty of carrots. It should bear the traces of the pine of the bay leaf and the piquancy of peppercorns, and be hearty with an abundance of onions, tomatoes, zucchini, turnips and celery.

Chicken soup can be munificent with marrow bones, laced with *lokshen* (thin noodles), crowded with chicken necks, generous with giblets, served with deep-fried mince *blintzes* (pastries) or, my personal favourite, chunky with chicken feet (only for advanced users). In its true and unrefined form, it ought, at the very least, to be bobbing with *kneidlach*.

Kneidlach are little dumplings made with *matzo* meal, seasoned with cinnamon and held together with eggs and a couple of tablespoons of *schmaltz*.

Ah, *schmaltz*. *Schmaltz* is a Yiddish word that doubles up for fat and the spongy cummerbund of flab some of us carry in the province of the gut. It is one of those words that is infinitely more tolerable in a recipe than as a personal descriptive noun. No matter how you prefer your chicken soup, it must be accepted that *schmaltz* in the soup, like stretch marks in motherhood, is part and parcel of the deal.

You don't need a degree in nutritional science to appreciate that there's a causal relationship, a dark desperate smuggler's contract between *schmaltz* in the dumplings and *schmaltz* on the thighs. And when you're aiming for svelte, *schmaltz* is the Osama bin Laden of foods. Matters would be greatly helped if there was a system of *schmaltz* identification, like caller ID, so that every time you put something to your lips you got a *schmaltz*-alert. But *schmaltz* is not in the habit of announcing itself. By the time you know about it, *schmaltz* is already happily in transit in your large intestine, planning where it would most prefer to set up home: *Hmmm, the inner thigh or the butt cheeks? Where are the better views?*

Because *schmaltz* is stealthy and sly, and has ways and means of wheedling its way into the most un-*schmaltz*y of foods, like sushi (the mayo, the avocado), you have to cross-examine the relationship between ingredients and the centimetres around your waist in the manner of US passport officers. Ignorance, according to the Food Fascist, is *never* an excuse. Ignorance is weakness. To lose weight you need strength. If I haven't cooked the food myself, I must make *schmaltz* assumptions and attendant enquiries.

Schmaltz, while obviously inherent in certain foods such as cheesecake and fries, is also the slow accretion of *overeating* and will creep up on you incrementally if you gaily consume heaps and heaps of healthy foods like fruit and hummus and salads with nuts and olives. There is an entire range of ostensible 'health' foods which have skulked into our psyches as gentle, unthreatening choices, but have done so under wolfish pretences. Muffins. Muesli. Granola. Health bars. Low-fat cheese. Apparently they're all doing secret deals with *schmaltz* under the table. They are, in fact, low-fat imposters and must be exposed. From here on in, I am to cultivate a deep and abiding suspicion of all food. All foods are guilty of *schmaltz* until proved otherwise.

Shifting the onus of proof in this way is a pirouette of personal agony. I am, by nature, a deeply trusting person and do not default into assuming the worst nor believing anyone is 'out to get me'. I know people like that and, come to think of it, they are skittish, edgy and ... skinny. Very un-me.

To help me keep a tally on what I'm eating, I have to keep a food diary. It's a detailed ledger of my weekly consumption, which exposes in no uncertain terms just how much I, to quote the Food Fascist, 'stuff into my mouth every day'. Allow me to confess that this remark induced in me a bout of late-onset self-revulsion for every occasion in which I'd swallowed anything without demanding a report card on the *schmaltz* content and exposing its treaty with the unbeautiful. It suddenly felt like a monstrous personal failing on my part to have eaten in ignorance. But there are circumstances. Invitations to dine out (so precious when you're a new immigrant). Meals in restaurants (when you can afford them, as a new immigrant). And who knows what bodily fluid might end up in your food if you're a difficult customer, particularly one with a South African accent? That joke about the waiter who goes up to a table of South Africans and asks 'Is *anything* okay?' would be hilarious if I hadn't personally overheard South Africans in restaurants. I'm trying to fit in here, not draw more attention to myself.

The Food Fascist had sensed my reluctance.

Would you rather be fat and polite or thin and bad-mannered?
Thin. I know the right answer to this question is thin.

Her instructions chafe against the very grain of my upbringing. My Granny Bee, who taught me all my table manners, was the soul of etiquette. She in turn learned everything from her mother, Doris, an elocution teacher who taught girls to faultlessly recite 'the rain in Spain falls mainly on the plain' when being able to do so apparently boosted one's marriage prospects. Barring suspicions of an ingredient to which one has a life-threatening allergy, my Granny Bee claimed that you *never* question the hostess about her food. Only a careless guest would fail to inform of existing food allergies when accepting an invitation. It's certainly not the time to bring up suppurating welts and anaphylactic shock at the dinner table, an indiscretion which could only result in a hostess's profound embarrassment at having catered inadequately. Best to eat up and head straight for the hospital.

This new eating plan is behaviour modification at its most unforgiving, pitting me against the tides of my upbringing and the soporific comforts of memory.

I lay out my white tablecloth for tonight's Shabbat meal and smooth its face of wrinkles. I stand the twin candlesticks my mother bought for me in the centre. I place the two plaited *challahs* I bought this morning from Wellington bakery on Bondi Road next to them. I do this because my mother did it, and her mother before her. I'm now the forerunner of a procession of women who either baked or shopped every Friday morning for this special Sabbath bread, and tradition has it that there must be two – one for Sabbath eve and one for the Sabbath itself. Despite a lifetime of insisting on my unique individuality, I am helplessly soul-stitched to this ritual of continuity.

Each time I surrender to these ancient habits, I'm tipped back into the cradle of times past to my mother's dining-room table, where I stand between my sisters, Laura on my left and Carolyn on my right, the Sabbath candles white and bright, the wine and the bread waiting to be blessed, and the smell of chicken soup singing sweetly from the kitchen. In the womb of that memory, chicken soup is followed by a roast (beef, lamb or more chicken), servings of vegetables, salads and then dessert, rounded off with chocolates and liqueurs. A Jewish meal is only complete when gastrointestinal rupturing threatens. There's no greater insult to a Jew than stingy helpings. Woody Allen describes one Jew talking about the food at a *barmitzvah*: 'Such terrible food... and such small portions...'

At my mother's table, 'being full' was never a reason to stop eating. Some of the many reasons to Have Some More included:

I cooked this especially for you because I know you like it.
You can't put so little leftovers back into the fridge.
It's freshly made.
I don't know when I'll find oxtail/duck/salmon fillets like this again.
You don't like my cooking?

Being full was, in effect, an insult. What sort of a person can't make room for a little bit more?

Refusing more was to snub the generosity and abundance that was on offer. Eating was proof that you were loved and that you knew how to love back.

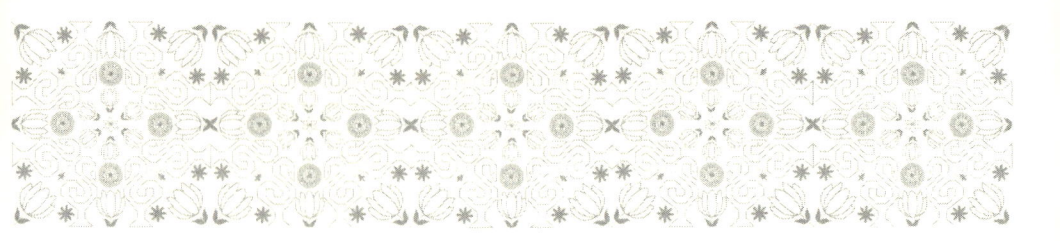

7
Grub

People show their character by what they laugh at.
GERMAN PROVERB

Jordan rushes into the dining room and asks, 'How long till supper?'

'Hours,' I say. 'Have an apple.'

'I don't want an apple, I want something salty,' he says, going to the cupboard. He riffles around for a bit and then says, 'Hey, what happened to all the chips and crackers?'

'I threw them out.'

'What?' he explodes. 'Why?'

'So I won't eat them.'

'They're not for you, they're for me.'

'If they're in the cupboard, I might eat them. If they're not there, I can't eat them.'

'But you're a grown-up!' He is patently disgusted with me.

How do I explain to my six-year-old that being a grown-up doesn't give you immunity from weakness, or the kind of tantrum that only a rabid appetite can throw? The first rule of self-discipline is: remove the opportunity. Nutritional studies reveal that we (in the first world) eat when it's there. Popcorn. Chips. Pretzels. Similarly, in our home we've always had a no-toy-gun policy (including water pistols or plastic swords) to engender a pacifist environment. I have noticed that the first thing Jordan does is raid the toy box at friends' houses and arm himself with every plastic piece of artillery he can get his hands on, as if he were setting off for a very brutal war. Lack of opportunity clearly doesn't kill desire. I wonder, shuddering, whether it in fact inflames it.

Jordan goes to the fridge and grabs three Granny Smiths – one in his mouth, one in his hand and one in his pocket. Much healthier than chips. I'm a mothering marvel – he just doesn't realise it.

'Is anyone coming tonight?' he asks.

I swallow. 'No, my darling, it's just us.'

'What about the Kahns?'

'They're busy tonight. They've been invited out somewhere else.'

The Kahns, Ross and Samantha (Sam) and their boys, David and Matthew, arrived in Australia from South Africa six weeks after we did. Ross and I knew each other from writing workshops in South Africa many years ago, but I'd only met Sam briefly once before. Sam, in what must have been a lethal cocktail of post-immigration rapture and jetlag, fell pregnant days after arriving in Australia, hence little Asha. Sam was the only other new immigrant I know who was as miserable as me – and sometimes even more so, given that she had pregnancy and then a newborn added to the lethal cocktail. She has the saddest, warmest hazel eyes that make one think RSPCA advertisements just aren't trying hard enough. Together we missed Africa without apology or restraint, on bad days listening to African music, reminiscing, holding hands and crying. On good days, she'd grab me to go for a walk along the beach or a skinny-dip at the Women's Baths in Coogee and coo, 'You can't do this in Johannesburg!'

When we first arrived in Australia, we were flooded with invitations for Shabbat dinners. Jewish geography is its own phenomenon, matched only by Jewish hospitality. Anyone who knew us – directly or indirectly, via the kosher grapevine – had us over for a Shabbat meal. In that first year, we travelled the length and breadth of Sydney on Friday nights. But after the flurry of 'welcome' invitations, people spend Shabbat with their own families, which is understandable as much as it is lonely for those without family. It's very easy to feel sorry for yourself when Shabbat beckons and there's no-one to share your chicken soup with. Without taking measures to fill the Shabbat gaps we'd always be a family alone. So Sam and I made a Shabbat pact: if ever we were alone, we'd do Shabbat together. Since then, most Friday nights we end up either at their place or ours, cobbling together whatever's in our fridges, making as if our children are each others' cousins, singing our Shabbat songs, including the rap song passed on to me by a friend's teenage son Raphael: 'S is for Shoibbos, H is for Happy Shoibbos, O is for Oy it's Shoibbos...' And I never see Shannon and Jordan as happy as when David is showing them the latest YouTube clip or they're climbing with Matt and Asha in their treehouse. But every now and then, one of our families is invited out elsewhere.

'I hate it when it's just us,' Jordan says.

Just Us. Shorthand for No Family, No Friends. And just like that, it swipes from nowhere. That terrible emptiness. That hollowness. The vacuum that's never been filled by the loss of my parents and sisters and the abundant life we had back in South Africa.

'Me too,' I sigh.

GRUB

'Aren't you having any?' Zed asks.

'No,' I say as I squeeze a sachet of miso paste into a cup of boiling water and sprinkle the skinny dust of dried seaweed and tofu on top.

'Surely you're allowed just a bit of soup?' he asks, eating his third thick slice of bread slathered in butter.

'She threw out all the chips,' Jordan quips.

'They're not healthy,' I say.

'Like McDonald's,' Shannon says.

'Nana always takes us for McDonald's when we're in South Africa,' Jordan says. 'You never let us have it anymore.'

'I know, I'm a real mean mum,' I say.

'I love Nana's chicken soup,' Shannon says.

'Yes, remember how we ate it in the middle of the night?' Jordan says, recalling the week of jetlag we endured on our last trip back.

'That was the best fun. When are we going to South Africa again?' Shannon asks.

I shrug. 'Some day.'

'A man came to school today and told us about witchetty grubs and bush tucker,' Jordan says.

'And he played the didgeridoo,' Shannon adds.

'Did you taste a witchetty grub?' I ask.

'No. Yuck. Dis. Gus. Ting,' Jordan says.

I have only the vaguest idea of what a witchetty grub is (something to do with Aboriginal culture) yet Jordan, at six, knows. At school my kids are learning all about Australian flora and fauna, leaving me lagging behind. Just the other day Shannon pointed out a slater to me. It took me a while

43

to realise she was talking about an insect. She knows her kookaburras from her lorikeets and while I run for cover, convinced it's an omen of Armageddon, she's perfectly at ease with a flock of flying foxes blotting out the sky overhead.

Zed watches me sip my miso. 'How's your watery dishwater fishy soup with bits of sea grass and bean curd?' he asks. Everyone laughs but me.

'I really don't like to be laughed at,' I say.

'We're not laughing *at* you, we're laughing *with* you,' Zed offers.

'I'm not laughing,' I say.

'You haven't laughed for four years,' Zed says sadly into his soup.

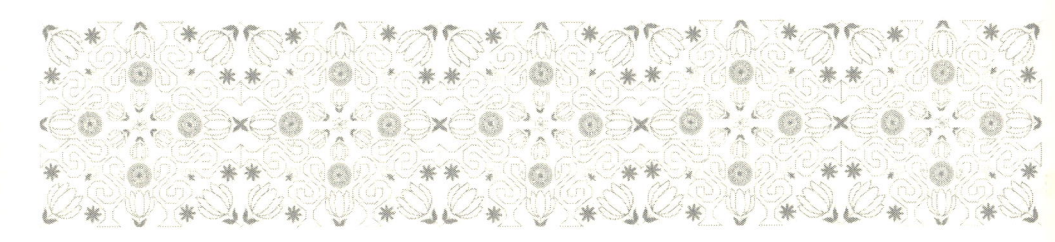

8
Shiver

On the tip of the tongue lies the fate of the entire world.
YIDDISH PROVERB

Zed's exaggerating. Of course I've laughed in the past four years – but rarely and probably not at myself. I don't find many things funny. I'm still getting the hang of the Australian sense of humour as well as that innate toughness that probably comes from being surrounded by all these poisonous arachnids and sea creatures that my children are becoming so *au fait* with. For the kind of girl I am – not the camping, outdoorsy, 'oh-there's-a-scorpion-in-my-sleeping-bag-ha-ha' type – the very idea that I have to share a continent with all these noxious creatures has taxed my generosity to the max. All it takes is something small and bristly for me to yell, 'Funnel-web,' and to usher Zed to the scene armed with a can of toxic chemicals where he proceeds variously to spray and stomp the shit out of the offending bug. Trust me, this is the only reasonable way to dispose of things that will poison you fatally with one miniscule nibble. The last time he pounded the hell out of a small black thing, we retrieved a bit of lint and hair gummed together from under his shoe. In my defence, it really did *look* like a spider from afar, and why take a chance?

I can't imagine I'll ever be one of those wide-brimmed environmental types who voluntarily pets a snake or finds anything about a crocodile beautiful, but maybe, just maybe my children will be. I can look on the bright side, but it's difficult on a Friday night when we're sitting alone around a Shabbat table. Not that I'm blaming Zed.

If it's anyone's fault, it's my grandfather's. If he hadn't boarded a ship in Eastern Europe bound for Africa in the early 1920s, Zed and I would never have had to leave it. But I can't very well get angry at my grandfather. For one thing, he's dead, and for another, he didn't have much of a choice at the time.

My father's father, Solomon Fedler, spoke English with a thick Yiddish accent. He ate bread as if it were cake, with grunts of guttural satisfaction. At the dinner table, he slurped his soup, sounding like those suction tubes dentists stick into your mouth so you don't dribble, which did a fabulous job of suppressing my appetite. My grandfather, whom I called *Zaide,* knew nothing of table manners. He was a poor Jew from Lithuania who fled anti-Semitism at the end of the First World War in search of a better future for his children. He ate like someone who knew what it was to be hungry.

When Zed and I contemplated immigrating, we did our research like the two legal academics we were, comparing the obstacles to entry into every English-speaking country and Italy – who'd mind learning a new language as long as it has words like *amoruccio* (my little love) and *fiori d'arancio* (orange blossom) in it? We evaluated the personal and professional requirements as well as the cost and indignities of various medical examinations (if you're from Africa, HIV is presumed until proved otherwise). We deliberated on the state of various economies in the short and long term, access to medical care and public schooling, taxes, the weather and lifestyle, levels of anti-Semitism (are Jews publicly lynched or just quietly despised?) and, very importantly for Zed, the sports played.

When he was alive, I never thought to ask my *zaide* why he opted for South Africa when there was Hawaii, Fiji and France (where apparently women don't get fat) to choose from. I might have been fluent in Spanish or Flemish or get all teary when the first notes of the 'The Star-Spangled Banner' strike up. I could've had that gorgeous Gabriel Byrne accent that makes people drift off in reverie imagining how you'd look with your clothes off in the early morning Irish mist. Instead, I instinctively say '*Voetsek!*' ('get lost' in Afrikaans) when I want to be left alone, '*Eina*' when I'm hurt, and I cry when I hear Zulu lullabies. Why did my *zaide* go for Africa? It's the arse-end of the world – until you contemplate Australia, that is.

Besides, it's not as if South Africa welcomed Jews in those days. Let's face it – if Jews were market shares, supply would always outstrip demand. There's never been a rush on Jews, even when other countries have been giving us away, like an 'Everything Under $1' table in Kmart. For reasons too complicated, painful and difficult to unravel in a book such as this, anti-Semitism is an inescapable phenomenon that, as a Jew, one learns to accept like I imagine the hunchback eventually makes friends with her hump. No use bitching about it, best rather to focus on a flattering wardrobe.

My relationship with my own Jewishness is as complex as any full-blown neurotic condition. There are wonderful aspects to Judaism, such as its rituals of blessing food before and after you eat, tithing one-tenth of your income to charity and taking a day of rest after a long week of work. But then there are practices that excite me very little, which invariably involve my exclusion based exclusively on my bosom. I am pained beyond articulation by the Holocaust, Holocaust denial, neo-Nazism and suggestions that all Jews belong at the bottom of the Mediterranean ocean. I can't imagine conjuring that level of hatred for *anyone*, let alone an entire race or nation. If it were up to me, Jews and Arabs would live harmoniously in the Holy Land side by side, like the Sneeches on Dr Seuss's beaches eventually did. And I'll never give up hoping someone will devise a cure for racial hatred and peace in the Middle East like they're working on for breast cancer.

But in the 1920s as the First World War ended, Europe wasn't a happy place for Jews, and there was a stampede to get out. With such a massive exodus, Jews quickly became like unsolicited mail where a little is more than enough and eventually everyone puts a NO JUNK MAIL sticker on the postbox.

After the US began limiting the number of Jewish refugees it would allow in, the South African government got nervous that it would be inundated with reject immigrants, so it did the same using the 1913 Immigrants Regulation Act which had been in place for years to prevent 'undesirable' people (mostly Indians) from entering. In 1921, the South African Secretary for the Interior instructed that this Act should be rigidly enforced against Polish and Russian immigrants, most of whom were Jewish.

Later in 1930, the Immigration Quota Act was passed, expressly limiting Jewish immigration to South Africa. A document entitled 'Immigration of Hebrews into South Africa' stated:

> One in every four who has entered the Union this year is a Hebrew, generally of a low type ... The European

population of the Union is small and every possible endeavour should be made to strengthen it and to ensure the quality of any additions to it, in order to preserve its position in relation to the hordes of native and coloured inhabitants. The existing conditions under which ... the better class of the European section is being depleted cannot be allowed to continue indefinitely without seriously affecting the standing of the European population as a whole. (State Archives, Pretoria BSN1/1/684 1 /60A)

Meanwhile, the Nazi aura was surfacing like a military migraine in Eastern Europe. To a Jew in flight, it made little difference whether a ship was headed for the UK or the US or Africa or Timbuktu, as long as it was a ticket away from pogroms. Fate turned on which ship company advertised in your *shtetl* or ghetto, what time of year it was, what restrictions or quotas were operating, who you knew, or whether you already had family in another country. South Africa seemed like a promising option – it was an emerging economy, not too industrialised or commercialised, where new immigrants could employ their skills and professions instead of being absorbed into sweatshops when they arrived. With the right connections and enough money to get started, a person could set up a new business and make a decent living. Lucky Jews who could secure papers and an escape from Europe arrived in Africa with hope in their bosom and Yiddish on their tongues. Despite all their cultural and religious idiosyncrasies, Jews were, after a good wash, white in a country where white was ultimately what mattered.

So my *zaide* wrote to a colleague named Zalman, who'd left for South Africa the previous year, asking if South Africa was the land of opportunity he'd heard it was. He waited and waited but a reply never came. What was wrong with Zalman – didn't he understand what a vital decision this was, one that would affect my *zaide*'s whole life? In the meantime, my great-grandfather encouraged his son to go and make a new life for himself. But what did my *zaide* know about South Africa? What opportunities or challenges awaited him? On a practical level, he couldn't speak a word of English. He'd also just married my grandmother, Chaya, and with money for only one ticket, he'd have to leave her behind initially to set himself up in Africa. But he had two *onkels* there who had promised him work.

Finally, apprehensively, he booked his passage.

On the day before his departure, while packing his suitcase, he came across the long-awaited letter from Zalman which had been intercepted by his father and hidden from him. And here's why: the letter painted a bleak picture for new immigrants in South Africa, detailing how tough it was to compete with cheap black labour, how impossible it was to get a job if one didn't speak English, and how the country was battling to absorb all the newcomers: '...*for those arriving now, prospects are not bright and no fortunes are foreseeable*,' he wrote. '... *it is not bright at all and therefore I feel as a duty to write to you before you have left.*'

Traumatised, my *zaide* confronted his father. Why? How could he have concealed this important information? His father shrugged and replied, 'What is done one cannot undo. I decided to destroy your colleague's letter but thought better of it. My intention was to forward it on to you once I heard that you were happy and all was going well. Don't worry, my son, farewell and God bless you.'

My great-grandfather understood all too well that knowledge has the power to dash the human spirit in a way that ignorance does not, and that if you are going to hell, it's probably better not to know.

The wheels of fate had already turned – a passage to Africa was booked. It was time for Solomon to leave. He said goodbye to his father, afraid he'd never see him again (he never did), shaken to his kidneys with uncertainty and drained of any optimism about his future in a foreign land it would take five weeks to reach, first by train and then by ship.

He boarded the train to Libau in western Latvia which would take him to London, crossing through Latvian territory, for which he needed a transit visa, valid for thirty days only. When he arrived at Yanishok, the Lithuanian–Latvian border, the Latvian train guards examined his documents and told him that his transit visa had expired the day before. My poor *zaide* panicked, not knowing what to do.

Suddenly, a man by the name of Mendel Melamed, someone he knew from his hometown, Zagere, appeared 'as if out of nowhere' and told Solomon to quickly give him ten dollars. Mendel then bribed the guards and Solomon was allowed through. It was a moment my *zaide* would often recount, saying it sent a cold shiver down his spine whenever he thought of it. Mendel Melamed had certainly saved his life.

When I think of this time in my family's history, I see heroes there: my *zaide* with his smallpox-ravaged skin and shock of red hair, who left his home and his father with so little promised and so much lost. And my great-grandfather who, with sacrificial compassion, deceived his son into a safe passage to a new world, certain that an unwelcoming Golden Land was better for Jews than Hitler's Europe. History would prove him right. Apart from Chaya and his sisters, the family my *zaide* left behind was wiped out by the Nazis. As was the brave Mendel Melamed and his whole family.

When Zed and I left South Africa some eighty years later, we too were blasphemous with doubt and numb with fear. But when I return to this story, like my *zaide* I too get a cold shiver down my spine, wondering if he'd gotten to the postbox before his father, or Mendel Melamed hadn't intervened with a ten-dollar bribe, whether I'd have been born at all.

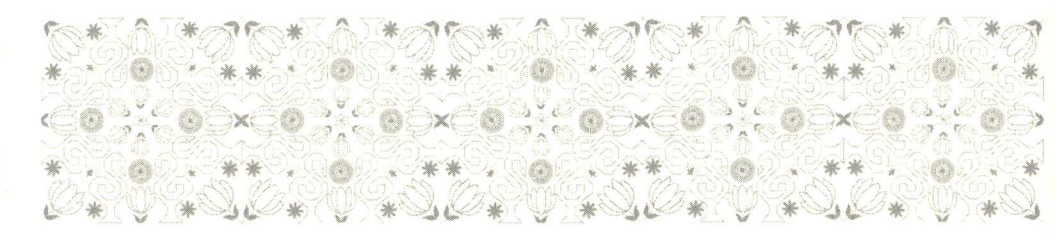

9
Reap

If you carry the egg basket, do not dance.
AMBEDE PROVERB

'I wish he'd never been born,' says Shannon, holding up a large scribble inside the cover of her Dr Seuss book. *My sister Shannon is fat and stupid*, it says.

'Come here *now*, Jordan,' I shout.

'Am I in trouble?' he asks as he shuffles into the lounge room.

'What is the meaning of *this*?' I ask, holding up the book for his inspection. He narrows his eyes and pretends to be reading it for the first time.

'How dare you call your sister fat,' I say.

'I'm not fat,' Shannon says, tears in her eyes. 'Mum's the one who's on a diet.'

'No-one should be calling anyone else fat in this house. It's a mean and hurtful thing to say. How would you feel if I called you fat and stupid?'

'Well I'm not fat,' Jordan says.

'What about stupid?' Shannon mutters.

'Enough! How dare you write in her book? That can't come out. It's there forever.'

'We could tear the page out,' Jordan suggests cheerfully.

'What about the first page of the story?' I hiss.

He shrugs and says, 'It's a stupid book anyway.'

'Right, that's it,' I snap. 'There are consequences for what you've done.'

'What sort of consequences?' he asks.

'I'll think up some horrible, evil punishment for you,' I say. 'Like no dessert for you after dinner.'

'That's so unfair,' he explodes, storming off. 'Why don't you just smack me?'

'There will no smacking but there'll be no ice-cream either,' I call after him. Actually, I should tell him he can't watch the footie match on TV tonight. That'll teach him. To punish effectively, the parenting books say, you have to find something that matters to your child. Punishment isn't punishment unless it really cuts into your child's very being or crushes his spirit, or something along those lines.

Shannon smiles the grin of the deeply satisfied – a Cheshire smirk two-fifths moral high ground and three-fifths sheer vindictiveness, eroding my confidence in the holistic value of this 'consequence-based' parenting technique I picked up during the excruciating four-week course in Positive Parenting I did a while back. I can't tell if I'm messing up the one child while getting the other one right, or vice versa.

'Logical consequences' is a great introduction to karma for kids. God is a tough one to sell given the tricky business of invisibility and I wouldn't want to *force* my kids to believe in Him given the whole freedom-of-religion human right in those children's conventions. But karma is such a sensible compromise, a halfway point for those who haven't made up their minds whether they believe in God or whether He's just a bunch of fairy-fluff and hoo-ha. Even if Shannon and Jordan turn out to be scientists like Zed's father without a mystical bone in their bodies, they can still handle karma which is essentially a mathematical formula: every action has a consequence.

Karma can get serious very quickly. I found this out years ago while on a two-month retreat at Hedgebrook writers' colony in the US state of Washington, working on my first novel. I'd been there only a few days, with vague nausea I assumed had something to do with US water. Maybe they didn't chlorinate it. Or use fluoride. Or maybe Americans only drink bottled water. But as two lines formed on a little wand in my hand after a big wee, karma thundered down on me as my mind caught up with what my body already knew. I did recall Zed asking, 'Aren't we sailing a little close to the wind?' the night before my departure. But I was going away for two whole months, and I just wanted one last night of rubber-free passion. Besides, I'd always dodged pregnancy bullets before.

But with two lines staring me down, I gained some overdue respect for the humble orgasm. Though not all consequences are as life-altering, body-distorting or relationship-testing as pregnancy, Buddhists actively live in that realm of careful consciousness. In Buddhism, every thought, every word and every deed is treated as a 'cause' setting in motion a boomerang-energy that will return. This idea I've sometimes heard expressed as: *As ye sow, so shall ye reap. You lie down with dogs, you wake up with fleas.* In the Jewish High Holy Day prayer book this is expressed as: 'Whoever digs a pit shall fall into it / the stone a man sets rolling rebounds upon himself.' That's karma, baby.

The way to create good karma (harmony, love, health), Buddhism suggests, is by making good choices (kindness, tolerance, self-care). When we make bad choices (selfishness, anger, closed-mindedness) we set bad karma in motion. Similarly, according to the Jewish mystical canon of the Kabbalah, good and evil have been mixed in the world since the time of creation, and it's our human responsibility to make choices for the good, which in turn separates good from evil. This 'repair' of the world is called *tikkun olam*. I'm charmed by the idea of all of us humans as little doctors of the world's spirit, healing, fixing and bringing it into harmony, except it's hard not to notice that we seem to be mostly polluting, hurting and destroying it, proving just how badly and sadly we've lost our way.

The simplest way to fill up on good karma or to choose wisely is to always ask: 'What are the consequences of the words, thoughts or deeds I'm saying, thinking or doing in this moment?'

In the quest for svelte karma, I'm often, of a lunchtime, poised at the crossroads between the custard tart and tabouli salad. Either way, there will be repercussions.

Karmic considerations are usually the last to spring to mind when you have a rumbling sensation in your belly and a packet of salt and vinegar chips in your hand. The consequences include:

A moment on the lips, a lifetime on the hips.

The food you don't eat won't make you fat.

To fortify me in these moments, the Food Fascist has provided me with a list of 'healthy alternatives' to all the foods towards which I naturally incline. Instead of chips, I can have ten rice crackers. Or an apple. Or four dried apricots. Or a low-fat yoghurt.

Invariably my body just about cracks up laughing at me (and you know how I hate being laughed at). 'Are you for real? A low-fat yoghurt? What planet are you from? Gimme salt. I want crispy. An apple? Ha ha ha!'

'What about an orange?' I offer.

'Shove that orange. Salt and vinegar chips! Salt and vinegar chips!'

I stall for time. I pour a glass of water and drink it down quickly.

'What did you do that for?' my body demands.

'Filling you up, seeing if you're thirsty. Hunger's easily confused with thirst.'

'I'm counting to three,' my body insists. 'One . . .'

I know my body well enough. Just like when Jordan has a tantrum, there's no point in getting into an argument. Ignoring a craving only compresses and intensifies its energy. Oh God, it could come back as a *binge*. Positive parenting has taught me this much: defuse. *Avoid a fight at all costs.* Though my body and I are on the same team, it just doesn't realise it. While it's yelling and carrying on and making a scene like an overtired toddler in the confectionary aisle at Woolworths, I just have to be the adult here.

I put exactly ten chips on a plate.

I sit down at my dining-room table.

I savour every bite as those sixty seconds on my lips transfer themselves to a lifetime on my hips.

'There, happy now?' I ask.

'More?' it asks.

'Nice try,' I say. 'It's tuna and lettuce for you for lunch.'

10

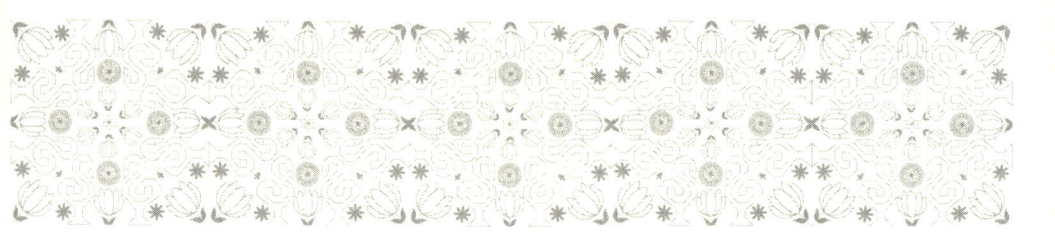

Greenhorns

The buffalo does not wander from the marsh where it was born.

NGABATA PROVERB, CONGO

By the time I was born, in 1967 on the cusp of spring, my *zaide* had come a long way since arriving in South Africa back in 1926 with his single suitcase and one glass eye, gained in an accident when he was sixteen on the night the First World War broke out. On his arrival, he'd been met by his two *onkels* who were disgruntled to discover he'd gotten married only ten days before he left Lithuania, muttering, 'A married man should stay with his wife.' Apparently while it was acceptable to exploit the labour of a bachelor, it wasn't done to exploit a wedded man.

Back then, he'd slept in an outbuilding while learning to read and write English, straining to understand what lambs' tails had to do with literature when his teacher suggested he get hold of Lamb's *Tales of Shakespeare*. He'd scrabbled pennies together, doing whatever work he could find, until he'd saved enough to bring my *bobba*, Chaya, out a year later. Some years after that he was able to bring his sisters to South Africa, making space in his modest home for one of them, Malke, who lived with him and *Bobba* Chaya for many years while everyone looked for a husband for her.

He recalled borrowing a few chairs and a table and making their beds on the floor. 'A life, a normality was beginning to take shape ... we bought [a few of the] barest essentials. A dream had materialized. We had a permanent "Home, sweet home",' he wrote in his autobiography, *Shalechet*.

Of this time, *Bobba* Chaya offers a different view: '*Our road was not strewn with roses / in this our beautiful land / we were greenhorns, foreign and poor / we had difficult times and were often forlorn / ... it is often just this [writing poetry] / that passes the time and suppresses the pain / for the people I so miss ...*' (translated from her poem, 'My Life').

Whenever they could, *Zaide* and *Bobba* took in newcomers, strangers who had nowhere to stay, and helped them get on their feet. Solomon supported a massive extended family for most of his working life, putting himself in debt to help his sister Malke and the man she married (at last!) to get started in business. Letters from friends in Lithuania begging him to bring over their relatives never stopped coming. He always did whatever he could, but stringent anti-immigration laws and bureaucratic obduracy made success scarce and he sometimes had to turn away from outstretched arms. The burden of constantly being asked to be a saviour weighed heavily on him. He was, after all, just an ordinary man, not a superman. He tried to bring his own father out from Russia but could never get permission from the authorities. He was even prevented from visiting his father's grave when he travelled to Russia in 1964.

Bobba Chaya spent her days writing poetry in Yiddish, laden with the agony of her separation from her family, the helplessness of distance, and her dreams of meeting up with her father and mother again. Her family was trapped in Europe though she and my *zaide* never stopped trying to get them out. But in the end, she was her family's sole survivor. She suffered a series of heart attacks and died just a few weeks short of her fifty-fourth birthday, proving with poignant irony that survivor guilt is enough to kill you.

By the time the Depression hit, Solomon had found his stride. He worked even harder, a battler to his marrow, and eventually started up his own printing business, Fedler & Co., which he was proud could offer employment to others. Like many Jewish immigrants, he made good in Africa. I remember him as a man with a great and generous heart, devoid of a single racist tendency, who wasn't afraid of a hard day's work and relished a little culture through the Yiddishe Cultural Federation.

Solomon's three children were born in South Africa in the 1930s, '40s and '50s into financial security and glorious weather, making these golden years for Jewish immigrants. In his later life, his children and ten grandchildren lived within a two-kilometre radius of his home. Even when he could no longer drive, he could still walk the few blocks to pop in for a cup of tea and a biscuit of an afternoon.

One spring Sunday morning he insisted that all his grandchildren gather in my parents' garden for a photo session. I wonder if he had some prescience of what was to come. Today, most of his children and grandchildren are scattered like seeds across the globe, in Toronto, Israel, the US and Australia.

I'm grateful that he never lived to see how many of us became the scatterlings of Africa. But then he, more than anyone, would have understood the exigencies of exile.

GREENHORNS

Pap and gravy have to be eaten with the hands. On the steps of the laundry to our big house, Violet, my nanny, taught me how to lift the *pap*, a porridge-like substance made from maize meal, with my middle three fingers, and dip it in the gravy, while scooping up some spinach to finish it off. I found the spinach bitter, though sitting with her I learned to love its bitterness because it came with freedom from Granny Bee's strict table manners of use-a-knife-and-fork, chew-with-your-mouth-closed and elbows-off-the-table.

I don't know if there's a word for 'obese' in Sotho, Violet's native tongue. But carrying a bit of extra weight around the tummy, thighs and buttocks in African culture is the mark of a well-fed, satisfied woman. Sitting alongside her, she always urged, 'You want more?' laughing a deep throaty chortle when I nodded, yes, please.

As a baby, I was carried on Violet Matlapeng's back while she did the housework. Like the children of many black South African women employed as domestic workers, her two daughters, Gladys and Nthabiseng, were cared for by her own mother in Bophuthatswana, one of the artificial 'homelands' invented by the apartheid system to disenfranchise black people. Violet never married and when I asked her why she always said, 'Ag Jo, men are too much trouble.' Violet looked after me, changed my nappies and sang me lullabies in Sotho.

At my Jewish day school, we sang both '*Die Stem*', the official Afrikaans South African national anthem and '*Hatikvah*', the Israeli national anthem. But it was Violet who taught me to sing '*Nkosi Sikelel' iAfrika*', the unofficial anthem of the oppressed people, and we'd sing it together while I helped her fold the big sheets, she lapsing into untutored instinctive harmonies. I ran to hide in her apron when my father lost his temper; and she smacked me with a wooden spoon on my bottom when I was rude to her. She brewed beer in her little backroom and sold it to the men who came and sat on wooden boxes in our backyard.

My family lived in the northern suburbs of Johannesburg, designated a Whites Only Area by the Group Areas Act of 1950, a fair distance away from the townships of Soweto and Alexandra where most black people lived boxed in shanties and shacks. The atrocities that took place far away from our high walls filtered down to us through the constipated reporting canal that was the censored South African press: children shot by police, people tortured in custody, prisoners falling out of windows or slipping on soap and cracking their skulls. We didn't know the half of it and the half we knew we didn't want to believe. Looking back, I wonder if innocence is sometimes a naiveté, a failure of the imagination to embrace what is confronting and uncomfortable. Perhaps ignorance is a wilful blindness. A fabulously convenient alibi.

In South Africa, Jews were part of the privileged upper and middle classes, relieved with our lot after our embattled history of persecution. A more charitable interpretation, perhaps, is that Jews didn't want to make waves or draw too much attention to ourselves. We were immigrants in a country that had been fought over by its African tribes and claimed by the Boers as a homeland. Apartheid was evil, but even as we knew it to be wrong we were immersed in it. Entrenched in it. Benefiting from it. To black people, Jews were just part of the rich ruling class, oppressors with *yarmulkas*.

There were Jews who joined the struggle to end apartheid like Joe Slovo, Ruth First, Helen Suzman, Arthur Chaskalson,

Raymond Suttner, Albie Sachs and others, contributing their work, vision and humanity towards ending the suffering of black South Africans. Because of people like them, I was sometimes proud to be a South African Jew. But for the rest, my Jewishness always felt compromised by my whiteness.

Every day my mother cut out my father's leader page cartoon from the daily newspaper, *The Star*, and stuck it in a big album. As one of South Africa's greatest political cartoonists, he's spent his life parodying the absurdities of apartheid. Every once in a while, the undercover security police came to check on him, to see whether the heart of a communist beat in his Jewish chest. But of Marx, my dad was only interested in the brothers Groucho, Harpo and Chico. He picked up a pencil at the age of four and fell into political cartooning because without Walt Disney or Marvel Comics to work for, what else was a boy with such a gift supposed to do? Dentistry? (Actually, that's exactly what my *zaide* had in mind for his youngest son.) He can't change a light bulb (not without a lot of whining) or remember where he's put his glasses (usually on top of his head), but what he can do in three minutes with a piece of paper and a pen proves that God does have His chosen few and that talent is a destiny.

I grew up clambering over the chaotic mess in his studio, which was Aladdin's cave meets pigsty, bursting with art books, Textas, canvasses, sketchbooks, paints and any bit of rubbish he'd managed to salvage in which he always saw great potential for puppets he'd someday build. *Ooh, keep that cork, match, bottle lid, pipe-cleaner, it'll make a great nose, sword, antenna, belt for an ostrich, rat, gladiator . . .*

Cartoonists are, of course, not real grown-ups. They're part-child, part-joker and part-prophet. They shout out whenever the emperor's willy is hanging out. Their job is to make people laugh, which I think is pretty revolutionary as far as life's purposes go.

My dad took us all to see *Superman*, the movie when it first came on circuit. For me, this marked a personal heterosexual turning point which presented as a feverish crush on Christopher Reeve in lycra. After that, I nagged my dad to get me a poster of Superman for my bedroom since he was always sourcing images to use as references for his cartoons. Instead, he painted one for me of Superman flying up, up and away. In huge block-letter text emblazoning the sky were the words: 'SUPERMAN LOVES JOANNE'.

After that, I didn't worry so much about Samuel Finkelstein.

11

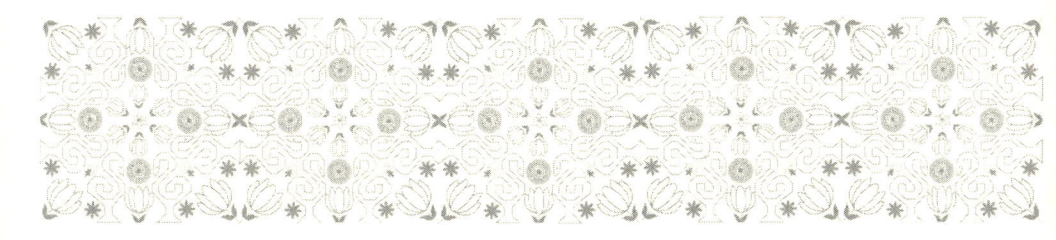

Rage

All is fair in love and war.
TRADITIONAL PROVERB

Superman, it turns out, was just the first in a long line of freedom fighters I've hero-worshipped. I can't think of anything sexier than a person with the conviction that the world is worth saving. Though in its absence, I'll grudgingly downgrade to a six-pack.

Ever since I was small, I worried about the world, mostly at night before I went to sleep. Apparently I was a 'sad, pensive and introspective child with an old soul', to quote an astrologer I once consulted who then had the gall to actually charge me for this depressing news. My parents had a name for it: 'oversensitive', invariably preceded with the suggestion, 'Stop being...' My mother tried to teach me to filter out the sadness, so as not to imbibe so much of it. But once I'd read 'Busload of children in India goes over bridge, twenty-three die' or 'Fire kills mother and child', I was a bundle of sobs and it was too late for the filter.

I cried easily (and still do) over accidents and tragedies that befell strangers, partaking in a vicarious grief I could never disengage as not my own. Bad news was sparingly passed on to me, the kid with an eggshell heart, on a need-to-know basis. When I rallied to raise money or knit blankets for disaster relief, my dad would sigh, 'You can't save the world, Joanne. Life isn't fair.'

It was easy to see his point. Unfairness in South Africa was inescapable and arbitrary, meshed into the fabric of every day. I didn't have to look further than Violet's life. She was separated from her family, living in a small room in our backyard some might consider too confining for an en suite, fated to do menial domestic chores for the rest of her life. I'd always fancied being a princess given the fabulous outfits, but the reality of having a 'servant' means repressing the awareness of the indignities they suffer while waiting on you. From early on, I hated my collusion in the whole warped picture.

When I was eight, Violet gave birth to another baby girl, Nthabiseng. I couldn't wait to get home every day so I could change her nappies and walk up and down our driveway singing her lullabies until she fell asleep in my arms. But one day I came home from school to find out that she was going to be sent back to Bophuthatswana to live with Violet's mother. I took the news like a hand takes being closed in a car door. It wasn't fair! It wasn't right! Why couldn't she stay? Violet was still breastfeeding her. She was just learning to walk and talk. I raged against the injustice of it. But Violet showed no emotion about the separation even though she might have cried herself to sleep in her backroom at night. She seemed to suck it up with stoic resignation and continued to iron and fold our laundry. And so she never got to see Nthabiseng take her first steps, speak her first words or lose her first tooth, though she was there in every family photo, cheering me on, when I did. I don't know of any way to feel better about this.

Then there was the unfairness concerning my sister Carolyn's hearing loss. It made me retchingly sad that she'd never hear ABBA's 'Fernando' or Queen's 'Bohemian Rhapsody'. Never. Did that mean her skin would never prickle the way mine did when I heard the music of *Les Miserables*? What would she do to pick herself up if she couldn't sing along to 'Walking on Sunshine'? The grief I felt about it was an edge I tried to stay away from, because it made me so heartsore that I didn't feel right listening to music if she couldn't. But every now and then I guiltily permitted myself a song or the Top 40 from behind a closed door in my room. I never wanted to enjoy the things she was denied, but I learned to love those things a little extra, to listen with that part of me that loved my sister too.

These inequalities I couldn't mend formed the basis of my ongoing gripe with a God who seemed to dish out good and bad fortune willy-nilly, a large scoop of health and prosperity here and a good glug of hardship and desolation there. My dad would try to console me by saying, 'If we knew why things happen the way they do, we'd be God. Let God rule the world.' Fair enough, but He seemed to keep getting things *wrong*.

My dad was right, though. Unfairness is part of life, like it or not. Suffering is inescapable, Buddhism tells us, and each of us must find our own way through the consciousness-shaping labyrinth of unfairness and make peace with it in the way that makes most sense to us. Some opt for a religious explanation ('*There is a reason for everything*', '*We can't know what God has in mind*', and so on); others give up on God entirely ('*No God would tolerate such unfairness – ergo, there is no God or if there is, fuck him*').

As a flick through World Vision pamphlets demonstrates, the big unfairnesses can tear your hopes to shreds. Thankfully there are also lesser ones to distract us. When we're not demented with outrage and a sense of crippling powerless about starving AIDS orphans in war-torn countries, we can become absurdly worked up over petty imbalances.

Right now, a full week into my new eating plan, I'm finding it easier to focus on the little inequalities. Like, for example, BMR.

BMR stands for Basal Metabolic Rate, which is, I've discovered, a silent metabolic player in weight loss. Metabolism is the rate at which the body processes food. Since you cannot see it, or feel it or watch it, unless you're a biochemist with access to a fancy laboratory and unflattering spectacles, you have to simply accept that it's there. Very much like God.

I always imagined food was a simple love affair between me and my plate, but there's a whole extended family bundled into the arrangement. I mean, who invited metabolism along to the party? Blood-sugar levels? Endorphins? Food has more connections than a celebrity on Facebook – hooking up with energy levels, bowel movements, moods, libido and immunity, just to name the inner circle.

The only sort of metabolism worth having is a fast one. Since it's responsible for chewing up the fat in your body, you'll want it to work like a sweatshop of illegal immigrants, after hours, weekends and overtime. But here's the real unfairness: everyone's metabolism is different. Like intelligence and good looks, it's mostly inherited. Men generally have faster metabolisms than women, another gripe feminism can add to its list of inequalities, as if vertical urination and world financial domination weren't sufficient. We each have to work with what we've got but, with a bit of effort, we can inprove on what we have.

Each person has a BMR that can be sped up with exercise. Another way to get it going is to eat – not a lot and certainly not *schmaltz*, but often. Every two to three hours. The worst thing you can do for you BMR is to starve it. Without food, it slows down. It forgets what it's supposed to do. It stops burning fat. There's no way to trick your metabolism; it's naturally suspicious. If you don't eat, like a Jewish mother, it assumes the worst – that starvation is imminent and it will hold every kilojoule in your body hostage, stockpile every bit of *schmaltz* and hoard for the lean times because it doesn't know when you're planning on eating again.

So if you skip a meal your metabolism will punish you for it. *This* is why crash diets never work. A week of celery soup can sometimes yield nothing but the same old blubber. So to keep your metabolism working, you have to keep eating and exercising.

But despite our best efforts, there's an inequality in the way BMR works. Some folk can cut down from four to three beers a day and lose two kilos in a week. I – can one stomach the injustice? – would have to cut out about six meals and chew sugar-free gum till I get salivary gland cramp to achieve the same result.

I believe this is what my father was trying to impart all those years back when he told me that I'd never be a model. What he meant was, 'You just don't have a model's metabolism'.

But what he also didn't know back then is that Carolyn would go on to become a medical pathologist with five university degrees. And that someday apartheid's walls would come tumbling down.

Life isn't fair, but if it were, there'd be nothing for the human spirit to strive for.

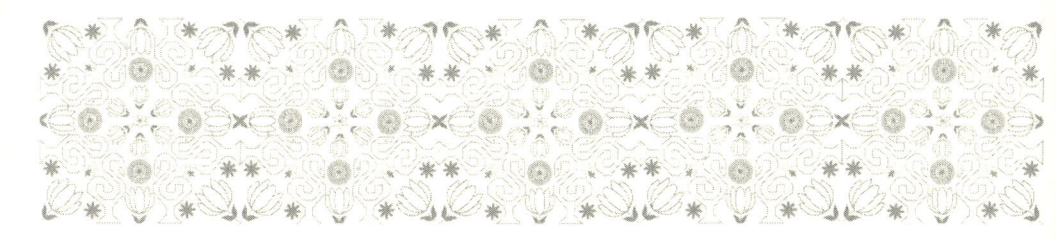

12
Convert

*All men have three ears: one on the left,
one on the right and one in his heart.*
ARMENIAN PROVERB

I was born a few weeks after my folks discovered what was wrong with Carolyn. My mother, in her anxiety to settle whether the child she was carrying was 'normal', wanted me induced and so I arrived two weeks before nature would have tossed me out into the world, which may account for the fact that I'm always early for an appointment or arrangement. Not two weeks, generally, but you can count on it being at least half an hour.

I was an early speaker (nine months, my parents say) and was the only one who could understand Carolyn before she started speech and hearing therapy. So I translated everything my big sister said for my parents at a time when I was only just acquiring language myself. From early on we had a deeper way of understanding each other, a connection that had nothing to do with words at all but something winding through us as sisters, a whisper in the blood – that affinity twins often speak of.

WHEN HUNGRY, EAT

An interpreter's job is to find equivalences, to convert from one dialect into another to make two ends meet. Given that I became something of an interpreter while I was still in nappies – which, you've got to admit, is a head start on those parents who stick golf clubs or violins in their toddler's hands with an eye to the future – you could say I have a natural flair for translations.

'What's all this low-fat yoghurt and lettuce doing in the fridge?' Zed enquires. 'Where are all my beers?'

'I had to take them out, they were taking up too much space,' I tell him. 'They're in the cupboard.'

'Beers don't get cold in the cupboard.'

'Yes, but yoghurt goes off in a cupboard.'

He contemplates the wisdom of my observation.

'Put a bit of ice in your beer,' I suggest.

'Spoken like a real beer drinker,' he says, sighing. 'I might just pop down to the RSL to get a cold one.'

RSL stands for Returned and Services League of Australia, having its genesis as a social club for Australian war veterans and the ex-service community. With branches in just about every Australian suburb, one can, of an evening, if one is a member as Zed is, go and play a game of bingo, get a steak, chips and cold beer all for ten dollars, and find yourself caught up in a raffle to win a meat plate predominantly involving various cuts of pig. There is no South African equivalent I can think of, for an RSL is a bit of a club, a dash of a casino, a few parts pub and a dollop of a diner all rolled into one. It's one of those quintessentially Aussie institutions that's difficult to explain to a non-Australian but one which Zed has embraced since we've been here. It certainly comes in handy of a Sunday afternoon when your wife has taken her empty stomach out on you and all your beers out of the cooler.

Recently, I've made some damn fine discoveries given my aptitude for conversions. They involve lettuce and low-fat yoghurt. Just as 'cheeky' might do as an English substitution for Yiddish's *chutzpah* or 'hospitality' for German's *Gemutlichkeit*, lettuce and low-fat yoghurt can be substituted for a whole orgy of high-*schmaltz* foods. Since cream, mayonnaise, and sauces are now all *verboten*, I've worked out that low-fat yoghurt, admittedly low on sex-appeal and taste, can be *tzuzz*ed up with a bit of lemon juice, garlic, mustard and a few chopped up chives. And ta-dah – you have a relatively exciting salad dressing, sauce or dip, in a *Queer Eye for the Fat Guy* kind of way. Because let's face it, what is a salad without the dressing (tasteless rabbit-feed), the chicken without the sauce (desperate and dry) or the crackers without the dip (Long Bay nibblies)?

For something sweet, I've been adding fruit pulp to yoghurt and, after some quiet time in the freezer, it converts into something close enough to ice-cream to give the tastebuds a reason to carry on.

This brings me to the lettuce, which with its large leafy surface area is a crunchy substitution for bread, tacos and wraps – and doesn't use up any carbohydrate allowances. In the past week, I've eaten lettuce hamburgers, sandwiches and rolls. The only thing lettuce can't be is toast. Trust me, it doesn't work.

Despite Zed's huffing, I refuse to feel guilty about claiming space for my low-fat yoghurt and lettuce. They're my new best friends and I'll heartlessly evict other foods from the fridge to make place for them amongst the litter of leftovers. This isn't an outlandish fetish, a fanciful dalliance nor an idle indulgence on my part. Day to day on my new eating plan is a practice of *survival*. This is Tough Love on the *tuchus*. I'm clawing my way from one meal to the next, thankful just to make it through without a binge or a fall from calorific grace. A week's careful preparation of skinless chicken breasts with salad, and oats with blueberries, can be destroyed in a moment's weakness by a mosey past KFC. Though an individual battle may have been lost to a packet of Kettle Chips, the war isn't over till the skinny lady sings.

Despite these successes, I can't claim gold ribbons in all events. There is, sadly, no translation for chips. Over the weeks, I've been experimenting with all sorts of low-fat rice crackers, especially salt and vinegar flavoured ones but, like a lover who just hasn't had enough experience, they fail to bring one to a point of satisfied completion.

I know this disappointment well. Since we've arrived in Australia, we've had plenty of practice searching for replacements for all we've lost. We've substituted the gas 'barbie' as the Australian version of the South African *braai* (which never delivers the smoky charred taste you want from burned meat, but starting an open fire on a hot day in Australia will get you arrested); we've made peace with under-flavoured sausages as a substitution for the peppery, coriander-rich *boerewors*; we've embraced Vegemite as the 'make-your-child-retch' equivalent of Marmite, and Zed has made the switch from Castle Lager to Victoria Bitter beer.

But no matter how hard you try, some things can't be translated, like *schadenfreude* in German or *nachas* in Yiddish.

Or grandparents in any language.

It's got me thinking that perhaps hunger is just an emptiness for the things that get lost in translation.

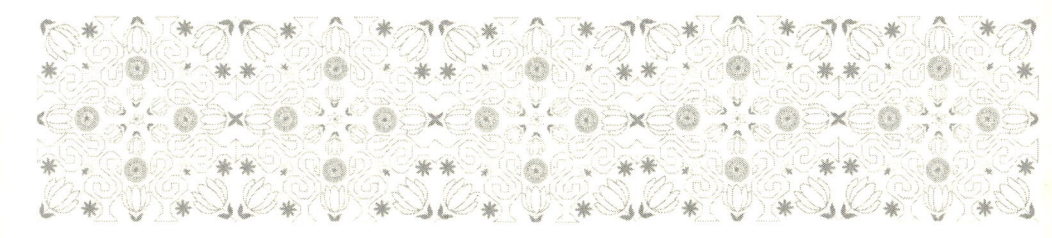

13
Scoff

Settling a dispute through the law is like losing a cow for the sake of a cat.
CHINESE PROVERB

By fifteen I'd ditched the lycra for kaftans and was into Gandhi, the vegetarian pacifist with cute glasses. With a brain as big as his mighty heart, he told the world that 'An eye for an eye makes everyone blind', which – no disrespect intended – makes God's retributive injunction in Exodus about eyes and teeth seem a little kindergarten. I felt in him a kindred spirit, certain no-one ever told *him* to stop being oversensitive.

Then in my late teens Nelson Mandela became my champion and, because love is probably blind as well as impulsive, I followed this righteous man who'd fought for justice and freedom into the law without making further inquiries.

Had I understood that law was less about fighting for lofty principles and more about cultivating arrogance and overcharging people, while encouraging them to pursue their miseries into the courtroom where they're sure to have their credibility and bank balances torn to shreds, I might have opted for flower-arranging or midwifery, genteel practices that don't induce ulcers or require a PhD in unpleasantness.

I'd always imagined law to be intrinsically bound up with sacred ideals like goodness, morality and, dare I say, God. And if you think I'm going too far here, remember how God told Abraham he'd save the cities of Sodom and Gomorrah if he could find just one good man? (You'll recall the fate of Sodom and Gomorrah – it didn't end happily.) Likewise, I challenge you to name anyone who's been through a lawsuit who wishes to repeat the experience.

Aha! See, that was a trick question – there are in fact no such people.

Sadly, law is not in the business of harmonious restitution or the righting of wrongs, but rather of protracting conflict and indulging the extravagant tastes of lawyers in French champagne and trips to Tuscany (not that I have anything against French champagne nor tourism to Tuscany, especially if they involve me).

I spent seven years in law school, two as a legal academic and a further two running a legal advocacy centre only to discover what a bleak and miserable profession the law is, a soul freezer. But then again, I was probably never cut out to be a lawyer, just like I was never built to be Australia's Top Model.

In law school, my eyes glazed over when my corporate law professor talked about 'debentures', a word I'd always associated with those gummy dental replacements my *zaide* kept soaking in a glass next to his bed. I made a habit of asking dumb questions like 'Was the accused male or female, black or white?' when trying to work out the legal solution. My professors reminded me (patiently at first, but with increasing irritation) that these were 'irrelevant' to the legal principle. A word of caution about people who tell you that the questions that press most urgently up against your heart are *irrelevant*: these people aren't to be trusted with the kind of world you'd like to live in. Most of the cases in criminal law featured African names. I heard it said by fellow students, more times than I can bear to recall, that this proved that 'blacks are more criminally minded than whites'. Why was apartheid's design in it all so difficult to see?

I admit these patterns distracted me from the legal principles, often grating against the grain of my being. But I lacked the language with which to explain myself. In this way, law left me hungry.

I once questioned a professor about a legal outcome in a torts case that left a destitute family even more destitute because their young son who'd helped bring in their income peddling wares had been electrocuted by a faulty wire whose maintenance was the responsibility of the municipal council. The family didn't qualify for compensation because, according to legal definition, the young boy had not been the family's 'breadwinner'. With a mixture of strained patience and regret, as one might pour a highly anticipated bottle of wine, spoilt not improved with age, down the sink, the professor said: 'Ms Fedler, you have the brains to be a brilliant lawyer, but not the heart.'

I'm all for a good laugh around a dining-room table but, if I can pick and choose, I most definitely prefer to be laughed 'with' rather than 'at'. One evening at a dinner party when I was in my final year of law school, a rather large partner from one of the top Johannesburg law firms asked what I was going to do after I got my degree.

'I'm going to be a human rights lawyer. Like Ghandi. And Mandela,' I answered.

When he finally stopped laughing *at* me he scoffed, 'If I were you, I'd focus on commerce-based subjects, otherwise no law firm will touch you. There's no such thing as human rights. Gandhi was deluded and Mandela's in jail.'

In my final year of law school we studied jurisprudence, the philosophy of law where at last it was permissible to ask questions like 'What is the purpose of the legal system?' And 'Is there such a thing as "natural justice"?' which, believe me, is as close to God as law school ever gets. Lawyers on the whole, are very loath to talk about God, which probably comes from the sensible division between church and state or perhaps, when someone gets around to doing the research, because they weren't breastfed as children.

But God wasn't always banned from legal discourse. All legal systems are derived from the ten commandments Moses *schlepped* down Mount Sinai. Who do you think started the trend of thou shalt not steal, thou shalt not murder? Even if God isn't your cup of tea, these are, at the very least, decent moral yardsticks for getting on with your neighbours.

But over history, Aristotle, the Stoics, Thomas Aquinas, Thomas Hobbes and Hugo Grotius (to name but a few) all fought over whether it was necessary for theology to be part of the legal equation or whether human rationality was sufficient. Hugo Grotius finally developed an argument separating natural law from divinity. And so – for now – God remains blanched from law in all shapes and forms, which I consider rather a pity since when people find themselves at the mercy of the law, this is when they need God the most.

As for where that leaves me, I can still admire the geometry of a perfect idea or the architecture of a well-constructed argument, just like I can a sequined cocktail outfit or a stained-glass-windowed cathedral. But as a short-nailed, flat-shoe kind of girl, I'm not overly impressed with cleverness for its own sake. I gave up strolls around the lake with spindly limbed literature for a trek up the mountain with hiking-booted law. I chose law for its grunt because, unlike poetry, I thought it could *do* things to change the world. I was sick with disappointment to discover that the Prevention of Family Violence Act was as effete and ineffectual (and far less lovely on the ear) as Yeats's 'Sailing to Byzantium', which at the very least makes your alveoli quiver with its beauty.

I'm also not trying to be provocative when I say the legal system is largely populated and controlled by white men and that this is not a good thing. If you're not a heterosexual white male you'll struggle to find your experiences represented in or understood by legal discourse. This is hardly an original critique of law, and brilliant academics have devoted their careers to showing how race, gender and economic factors burden women, minorities and people of colour; and steal their equality in a system that doesn't know how to handle difference. For example, Helena Kennedy's book *Eve Was Framed* exposes the sexism of the English legal system, and Patricia Williams's *The Alchemy of Race and Rights* does the same with race in the US legal system. You should feel free to go and look them up and read their work, but if you, like me, have a thing about unfairness, I'm warning you, it'll grate you up the wrong way.

This probably explains why in law school, I always felt like the fat girl at the party, watching from the sidelines, wondering why no-one ever asked me to dance.

14
Laurels

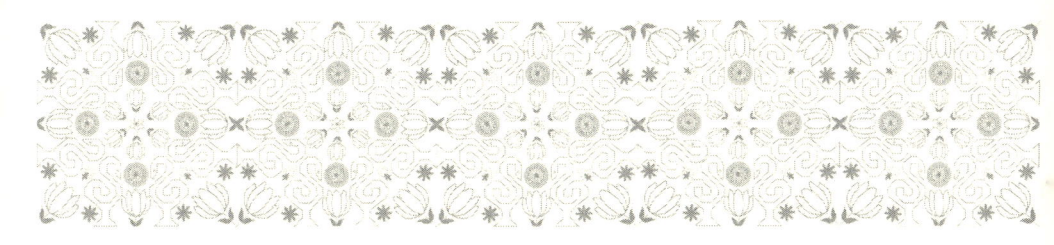

Who is brave enough to tell the lion that his breath smells?
BERBER PROVERB

'Do my thighs look big in this?' I ask Zed, turning around to show him my bottom. We're heading for the beach and I'm wearing a pair of board shorts. They're tight on me. There will be chaffing. Of course I won't actually get into the water. I hate cold water, which makes me the only wuss in our family. Beach excursions are never for *me*. For one thing, I have an uncomplicated antipathy to sand and, environmental sentiments aside, I agree with Zed that 'all beaches should be paved'.

No, I endure beach excursions because the children love them. They love the way you can roll around in sand and get it everywhere, into every bodily crevice and orifice. They love the waves that crash down on them as I'm wincing from the shore, torn between rushing for a lifeguard or giving it another few seconds for their heads to pop up through the foam. They love the ball games Zed plays with them in the water.

They plain love every bit of the experience that is the beach excursion. And what sort of a criminal mother would I be to deny them the pleasure of the great outdoors where you can get sunburn, sea-lice in your bathing costume, sand in your picnic and stung by bluebottles all in one afternoon?

Whenever we're on the beach, where you get to see humanity in all its contours, dimensions and uninhibited glory, Zed invariably reaches for his phone to call his friend Charles in South Africa. Charlie has a belly that approximates a nine-month pregnancy. Charlie eats and drinks like he's doing it for charity without fear of consequences since he has a freakishly healthy cholesterol coupled with low blood pressure. Their agreement is that Zed will call him every time he sees someone more corpulent than him. Zed doesn't use the word 'fat', though. What he says when he calls Charlie is, 'Hey Charlie, I've just seen a guy who's a couple of pies ahead of you.' And then the two of them spend half an hour discussing South Africa's performance in the latest rugby or cricket test matches. It's an astonishing friendship because if any girlfriend of mine called me up with such news, I'd tell her to have a nice life.

Even though I don't actually swim, I still have to dress for the beach. Which is why I'm in these shorts and this boob-binding, body-hugging top. I catch a glimpse of myself in the mirror and I'm positive Superman could most certainly not love me. Besides, I was never in love with Superman, it was Christopher Reeve. And look at what happened to him. There's a horrible twisted irony in Superman becoming a quadriplegic. I really hate what God did to Christopher Reeve.

Zed in his Speedos pauses at my question. He inhales and cocks his head to the side.

'It depends what you mean by big,' he says. 'I like big.'

LAURELS

I'm sitting in the Food Fascist's waiting room. It's my first weigh-in since I started this eating plan last week. All I've had today is a skinny coffee without sugar, a poached egg and some boiled mushrooms. To make a dent in my two litres of water daily, I've also drunk four glasses of water which are just announcing their arrival at the terminal in my bladder, even though I weed three times before I left home. How do koalas do it? Apparently they don't drink much water. Shannon told me the other day that koala is Aboriginal for 'no water' and that these tree-dwelling marsupials get most of their hydration from their exclusive diet of eucalyptus leaves. I can't really relate to a temperament that doesn't at least want to experiment with a range of foods, but then again, I'm pretty sure out in the wild there are no obese koalas.

On the walls of the Food Fascist's waiting rooms are a series of charts and posters I suppose could count as affirmations.

There's one about 'How to Enjoy Yourself in a Restaurant', with suggestions about what to avoid and what you can enjoy 'guilt-free'. There are also pin-ups about heart disease and diabetes and other conditions all rooted in the gusto of gastronomy the Food Fascist would have me believe is a pathetic personal weakness.

The door to the Food Fascist's office opens. A woman who's clearly been crying emerges, patting her face with a tissue.

My urge to wee becomes diabolical.

'Come in,' the Food Fascist says to me, unsmiling.

'Who me?' I ask dimly. There's no-one else in the waiting room.

'Good girl,' she says matter-of-factly.

I'm standing on her scales and I'm 560 grams less than I was a week ago. A drop in weight! I feel positively anorexic.

'Half a kilo a week is good going,' she says.

Is this . . . encouragement?

'Now, don't rest on your laurels, keep it up,' she says scanning my book of entries. 'What does this mean, "*Lots* of salad"?'

'Well, I went to a friend's house for dinner and, instead of having the lasagne, I just had heaps of salad.'

'No need to eat heaps of anything. You're not eating for the entire dinner party, just for yourself.'

I feel like a toddler who made it through a week without nappies but has just wet herself.

'And I see you only did forty minutes of exercise two days ago.'

'Um . . . yes,' I confess. 'I . . .'

'I'm not interested in your excuses. You want to lose weight, you need to do at least an hour a day.'

I nod.

I thought I did lose weight, but I'd rather chew my own tongue than point this out.

I barely make it out of her rooms without wetting myself and head straight for the ladies where I wee out what surely must be another whole kilo of urine. I then call Zed on my way home to tell him the wonderful news. 'These grams are dropping off me like flies.' I'm going to be thin, I'm going to be thin.

I feel faintly imbued with the miraculous.

Part Two

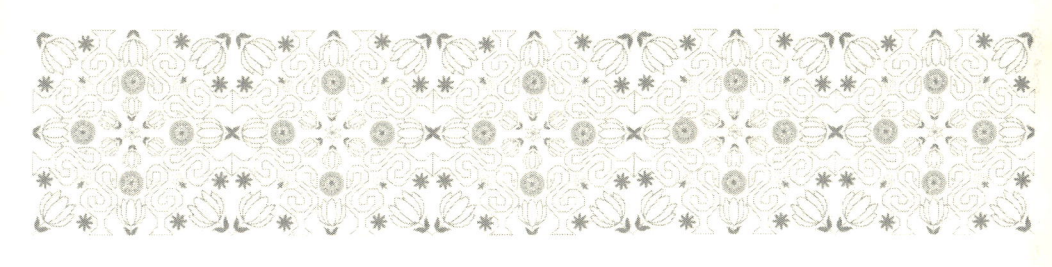

Hope

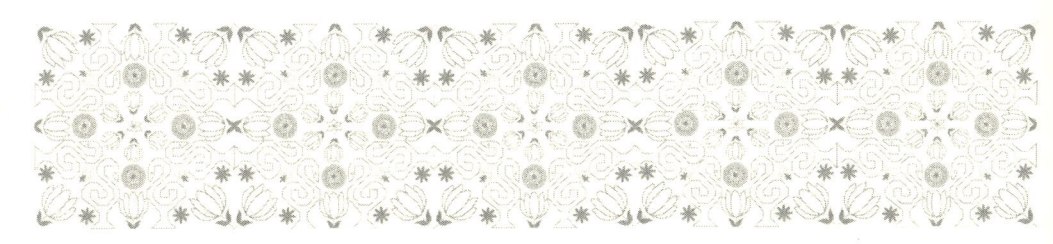

15
Cracks

May you live in interesting times.
CHINESE BLESSING

Is it just me or does everyone hope to someday witness a miracle? I'm not fussy – Moses parting the waters; Jesus healing the sick. Something you don't get to see every day, not so much for the spectacle of it but because of how it might change one's sense of what's possible.

I'm a bit of a gusher at the best of times so if I witnessed a genuine miracle, I'd probably run around shrieking, 'Oh my *God*! Did you just see that? Shit! Crikey! Can you believe what just happened,' almost certainly violating miracle-protocol, which I'd imagine calls for sacred composure.

Discounting the births of both my children – where I didn't run around shrieking on account of the epidural and the entrails I'd have been forced to drag around with me – I've never been present at a bona-fide miracle. But the events that unfolded in South Africa over the course of my lifetime were, in their own way, quite miraculous.

As a child, I knew we weren't living in joyful times. I'd eavesdrop on conversations around the dinner table while my dad discussed his latest cartoon and saw, even through the cataracts of childhood, how despondent my parents became after every election the Nationalists won. I never heard when the young Hector Petersen was shot dead in the Soweto uprisings in 1976. Nor was I told of Steve Biko, the young Black Consciousness activist, who died a year later in police custody from head injuries. Becoming politicised is a form of historic literacy which I only began to acquire many years later when I was at university and began to fill the gaps in my own history. I met people like my friends Zakes and Brandon, ANC Youth League activists who patiently educated me. Both Zakes and Brandon's older brother had spent time in solitary confinement for their political activism.

But in the 1980s, events around us hotted up politically and spilled into the classroom. There were a few lefty teachers at my Jewish high school who bent the curriculum to make the connections between the suffering Jewish people had endured in the past and the suffering of black people in South Africa, and taught us to ask the hard questions.

In 1982, activist and author Ruth First (the wife of Joe Slovo) was killed by a letter bomb. That same year Dr Neil Aggett, a prominent labour leader who tried to bring unity to the South African trade union movement, was found hanging in his cell after being detained by security police. In 1985, Botha gave his famous 'Rubicon' speech, in which he warned the world 'not to push us too far', and barked that South Africa would not give in to hostile pressure and agitation from abroad. It wasn't a time of great national pride. Botha was like an embarrassing parent you just wished would shut up.

These were 'interesting' times, but like 'interesting' people, it was impossible to predict which way things would go under pressure. When I started university in 1986, the cracks were starting to show as student politics began to encroach into academic studies. Mixed-race couples paraded around proudly, defying the Immorality Act, one of apartheid's little gems which forbade interracial sex. On weekends, I taught Shakespeare to students from the townships who were being educationally starved through Bantu education. I've never since come across the appetite for knowledge I witnessed in those hungry faces all desperately reaching for the golden ticket of a university pass. These kids, who studied without electricity and shared a shack with large extended families, were just so darn happy if you cared enough to show up. There was brightness there in eyes I've never forgotten, gratitude – for an intact textbook, or an extra worksheet – that choked me.

On-campus student rallies were more and more often decreed politically 'undesirable' and stormed by the security police. If you were in the wrong place – too close to the front, too near the edge, you might get a taste of tear-gas or be arrested. The adrenalin of those times was addictive. To care that much about anything is thrilling; fighting for something together with others sharpens your sense of purpose in the world. It enlarges you as your own ego merges with a tribal energy, like single voices rising in harmonies, in a symphony of human aspiration. Those university years were like the first rush of lust in a relationship. You can become addicted to the passion, spoiled for ordinary life which by comparison feels bleached of meaning.

Towards the end of the eighties, as the political contractions became more intense, we knew *something* had to happen. In 1989, PW Botha suffered a mild stroke (God's small contribution) and resigned the leadership of the Nationals' party which was taken over by FW De Klerk. De Klerk then went on to release Walter Sisulu, the former ANC secretary-general, and six other ANC leaders from prison. While the Berlin Wall was coming down, the walls of South Africa's apartheid were crumbling as if the earth was shaking itself free of partitions.

I was driving home from university on 2 February 1990 when I heard on the radio that De Klerk had unbanned thirty-four organisations, including the ANC. Political prisoners were to be released and all regulations on the media we'd grown so used to, were to be lifted. When friends and I watched Nelson Mandela walk out of prison on 11 February 1990 as we sat crowded around a small-screen television, we *knew* we were witnessing a miracle or something close to it, each of us lost in awe in a silence so perfect you'd swear the earth had paused on its axis in deference.

One of law's jobs is to maintain stability, which if you think about the four legs of a table, or a supportive bra, is not a frivolous endeavour. To keep society running smoothly, things must continue to be done the way they've always been done. This repetition builds tradition, custom and ritual, but also inspires law's bad habit, known as 'precedent'. By law's reckoning, certainty (even if it's unfair) is better for society than vacillating justice. It's the legal equivalent of staying in a crap marriage for the sake of the kids.

Up until this time, racist laws under the South African Westminster legal system could never be challenged by the courts because of a legal presumption that the legislature had not *intended* to be unjust. (Apartheid was riddled with these infuriating fictions that could make a sane person chew their own arm off.) Some of these included the Native Land Act of 1913, which prohibited black people from owning land, and the 1923 Urban Areas Act forcing black people working in cities to live in designated areas. But over this time, the South African legal system was shorn of its foundation and a constitution with a Bill of Rights took its place. The Constitutional Court was set up with a bench of anti-apartheid lawyers, activists and academics to be guardians of our future. All that ancient doddering precedent based on Roman law (whose property system included ownership of slaves) was scrapped.

Our new point of origin or *Grundnorm* (so named by the European legal philosopher Hans Kelsen) from this time forwards, given our appalling track record in this regard, was the right to equality, a notion that changed ownership, contracts, rape law, the rights of the accused – everything. Every area of law was to be illuminated with human rights. Something beautiful was happening and I could see my part in it.

So, to the smug law partner who scoffed at me all those years ago: Who's laughing now?

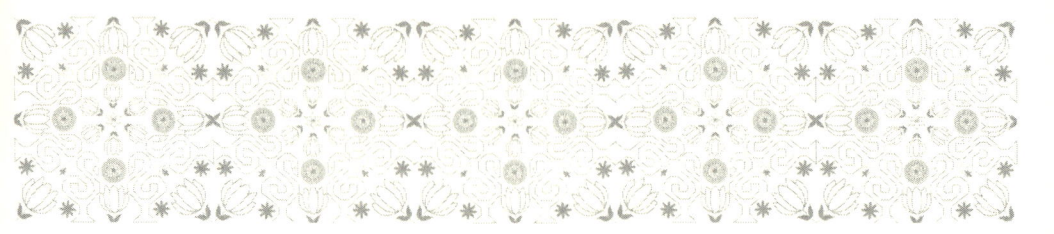

16
Banana

Prevention is better than cure.
TRADITIONAL PROVERB

'Have you got a jumper?' I ask Shannon.
'It's not cold.'
'Take one just in case.'
'Muuuuum,' she sighs. 'It's not cold.'
'What about a raincoat?'
'It's not raining.'
'In case it rains later?'
'No, I don't.'
'Well?'
'I'll just get wet,' she says.

I'm running out the door to try to get the kids to school on time and bump into Miriam, our elderly neighbour who lives in the building next door, who's shuffling off down the driveway to play bingo at the Hakoah Club in Bondi for the day. We shout our 'Hello Miriams' to her and she looks up vaguely, managing a small smile and a wave. I'm juggling bag, keys and ... what's this? A banana? Handling this banana in my overloaded state makes my deft and swift departure decidedly unnifty and sluggish (dear God, there's that word again). As I check Shannon has her saxophone and Jordan his school cap and excursion envelope, I wonder vaguely what this banana is doing on my person. It hasn't been more than half an hour since I had my little bowl of Special K and low-fat milk. It didn't adhere to me by vegetation levitation or follow me like a stray cat. I must have picked it up, though honestly, I don't remember doing so.

Madness is perhaps not the worst human affliction – some of the most inspiringly creative people are a little unhinged. The actor Robin Williams said that we've all been given a little madness which we should do our best to hold onto, or words to that effect. Albert Einstein defined insanity as doing the same thing over and over again whilst expecting different results which, come to think of it, may shed some light on my weight problem.

As I inch through the parking lot that is Sydney's work-run traffic, with a medium-sized, perfectly ripe banana nestling on my thighs, it slowly dawns on me that if I really want to transform my body, I'm going to have to fundamentally change my relationship with food. Whatever principles have guided me in the past have clearly not served me well. I need a new *Grundnorm*. This very much begs the question: what has my previous unidentified *Grundnorm* with food been all these years? Why do I eat? When do I eat? How do I eat?

The culprit, of course, is getting warm on my lap.

If I think about it – which I am consciously doing for the first time – my mother has for as long as I can remember always insisted, 'Take a banana,' no matter whether you were going out for an hour, on a long car journey or flying overnight. 'Take one just in case.' Just in case of what? In case (God forbid) you get hungry. So I've always taken a banana. Bananas are filling and are rich in potassium, not that I have the foggiest idea why this might be good for me. For all I know potassium might cause warts. Or kidney stones.

I always take a banana, and I always end up eating the banana. If you don't eat the banana, it gets bruised and mooshy and ejaculates in your bag, leaving behind a nauseating squished fruit odour that detergent cannot budge. Unlike apples and oranges, uneaten bananas don't take well to being recycled again the next day. Ethically speaking then, not eating the banana is also wasteful when there are so many hungry people in the world. I think I've eaten more bananas in my time because other people are hungry than because I am.

And there it is. The *Grundnorm* of my relationship with food: I have, it appears, always eaten so that I won't get hungry. If I suspect I might get hungry at some point, I eat to pre-empt that prospect. Hunger always gets shoved away at the front door like a Jehovah's Witness, never getting a chance to make itself comfortable, like an old friend, in the lounge room of my belly. Hunger, like rats and termites, has always been the kind of affliction against which one must take preventative action.

It would be hard to deny that my 'just in case' affliction affects more than just my eating habits. When we left South Africa, I packed every last paper – including all my files from university days, every love letter, every scribble (whether intentional or random) Shannon had ever drawn to take with us. I insisted on bringing the stone angel and birdbath from our garden, which had to be specially encased in wooden frames, as if Australia didn't have garden statues I could purchase on my arrival. No wonder we were 'overweight', filling up one and a half containers that needed to be shipped across the ocean. I've never understood the notion of 'travelling light'.

What if you get to your destination and find they don't have a hair-dryer, or a toaster, or a hot water bottle? Then you'll be sorry you didn't end up taking one just in case. Better to take them with you and be prepared.

Zed (as if to make a point) owns very little – by choice. He regularly sorts through the few items he owns, because apparently as soon as his neurotically neatly folded pile of t-shirts reaches the excessive number of five, he feels 'burdened' and needs to pare down again. It could be an unconscious passive-aggressive response to my mess, though he pointed out that he was like this long before he met me, but if I want to take credit for it, he suggests, 'It's all yours, baby.'

I remember an African–American musician I sat next to on a flight back from the US, after my year of study there, who helped me put my absurdly heavy backpack in the overhead carriers, saying to me, 'Girlfriend, why do you carry the world on your shoulders?'

He sounded just like my dad who once told me the parable of the Buddhist monk who's walking with his disciple when they come to a river. There they find a beautiful young woman who cannot cross. Without a word, the old Buddhist monk puts her on his back and takes her across. The two, master and student, continue along their way for hours, when the student can no longer contain himself he bursts out, 'Master, how could you touch that woman? Have you not taken a vow of celibacy?'

'Yes, but *I* left her behind at the river,' the master says.

Oh, how I'd love to be able to leave things behind, and to have the spiritual metabolism of a Zen master.

When I've read historical accounts of Jews who were evacuated during the Holocaust, I try to imagine being told to pack all my belongings into one suitcase or as much as I can carry on my person. How would I choose what to take and what to leave behind? Would sentiment or pure market value drive these decisions? And do objects become more or less precious at such times? These hypotheticals make my head ache, which is why I always carry painkillers.

Maybe I'll ask Miriam when next I take her some chicken soup. She's a Holocaust survivor – of her family of fifteen siblings, only she and two brothers survived. She told me this one day with tears that sprang into her eyes as if the anguish was as fresh as yesterday's grief. Miriam, now a widow, lives alone at eighty-six, with arthritis in every bone in her body, yet despite this pain she walks to the bus stop every day to catch a bus to play bingo. Without it, she once told me, she'd go mad. 'It's the loneliness, you see.'

We had kept passing each other in the street for months before one day she wished me a happy *Chanukah*. Until then I hadn't realised she was Jewish. After that I started sending her chicken soup, as one does. Now and then I see her struggling to empty her postbox because of her height. 'I'm shrinking,' she told me the other day, describing how she, with her arthritic fingers, had to take up the hem on her dressing gown because she keeps tripping on it. Whenever I help her retrieve her post, she asks, 'So, any love letters?' I once got a peek into her kitchen cupboard and, judging by the number of packets of quick-and-easy *kneidlach* and prunes she has there, the just-in-case principle may in fact be a Jewish trait. Jews who've had everything taken away suffer from terrible anxiety about never having enough, stockpiling food and other household essentials.

Perhaps I can claim this as an ancestral hangover?

But no. Who am I kidding? Even if I've inherited this neurosis, rather than single-handedly acquired it, it's become a convenient excuse. It may even be a bona-fide personality flaw. I just can't keep holding on to things for fear of not having. I hate not having what I want; like when the air stewardess says, 'We're out of the beef, would you like the fish?' 'Going without' ruins my flight, though as Zed is quick to remind me, 'Having the fish might be an inconvenience. *Crashing into the ocean* would ruin your flight.'

Maybe, as Shannon's teaching me, there are worse things than getting cold if it clouds over, or wet when it rains.

As I accelerate through an amber light, I realise that I'm going to have to start somewhere different in my new relationship with food. I can't keep taking the banana and eating it just in case.

From now on, I'm going to eat only when I am hungry.

But how will I know when I'm hungry? Does hunger present as a strident shrill shriek in the middle of the day, panicking one to excessive pastries? Does it creep up like a nasty rash, starting on the elbow then spreading everywhere? Is it like tinnitus, an almost imperceptible whine in the middle ear, never ceasing its pitch, which you have to simply train yourself to ignore?

I honestly don't know.

'Anyone want a banana?' I ask Shannon and Jordan.

'No thanks, I'm not hungry,' Shannon says.

'Yuck,' says Jordan. 'Dis. Gus. Ting.'

In this moment I am so proud of Shannon. She's not hungry and she knows it. I, on the other hand, must learn my own hunger. I am strangely illiterate in its language.

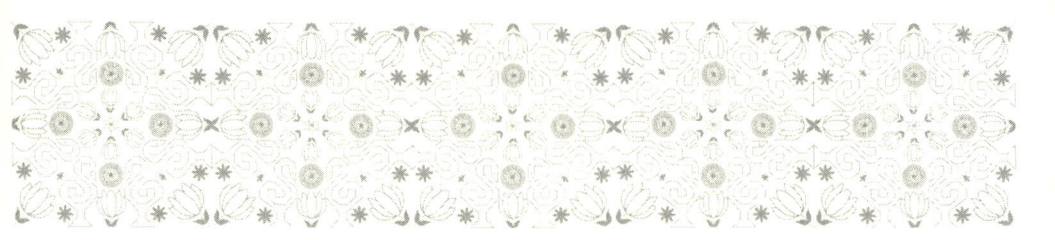

17
Blue sky

Strive to be a person who is never absent from an important act.

OSAGE PROVERB

I left South Africa in 1992 to study in the US on a Fulbright scholarship to Yale, with a banana in my overnight bag for the flight.

That summer I turned twenty-five and had buns of steel from years of Jane Fonda workouts and big dreams for my future as a human rights lawyer. In that pre-Clinton era, New Haven was muggy, everyone was single, and pizza-eating competitions followed tequila parties night after night. I spent long hours in the old law library reading up on theories of justice, and hopped on the Metro North into Manhattan whenever I had free time.

Yale was academically thrilling but it was icy cold through the snowy winter, and lonely for a girl so far from home. While smart, tense people were finishing papers and studying for exams, South Africa was on the brink of a new era. My fellow students weren't particularly interested in what was going on in a little country in the southern hemisphere fighting for its soul, not with all the reading material that had to be covered. After the fire and camaraderie of the years on campus in South Africa, Yale was cool and dispassionate, an Ivy League iceberg.

On 10 April 1993 when Chris Hani, the head of the South African Communist Party, was assassinated, I tried, through my tears, to explain to my Scottish room-mate Bonnie why I was crying. Hani had been one of the truly good men in South Africa and *didn't she see* we needed every good person to pull off a peaceful transition? Instead, sweet Bonnie offered to take me for a Ben and Jerry's ice-cream to 'take my mind off things'.

The predictions of 'civil war' and 'bloodbaths' terrified me – so many South Africans had already died. Yet Mandela and Archbishop Desmond Tutu were speaking only the language of forgiveness and peace, envisioning a miracle. At night I prayed for their safety – *Dear God, look after Mandela and the Archbishop, help them to lead us to peace . . .* – scaring myself with just how deeply and personally I wanted this.

Later that year Mandela and De Klerk were jointly awarded the Nobel Peace Prize 'for their work for the peaceful termination of the apartheid regime and for laying the foundations for a new democratic South Africa'. As we inched closer to democracy, I began to lose something. I felt lighter than I'd felt in years, maybe ever. My shame at being a white South African slowly lifted like a migraine that's finally been properly medicated. I'd never warmed to that concept of 'national pride'. Until now. Goddammit, we were going to show the world how it was done.

Despite the lightness in my heart, I came back from Yale big. I'd put on ten kilos over nine months in New Haven through a staunch regime of no exercise, late-night poring over legal texts and an exclusive diet of Ivy League canteen food – which was, just like every other university canteen fare, gratuitously oily and entirely loveless. I was also bloated and plumped with America's garrulous buoyancy and super-sized visions.

Back in South Africa, the ions of change filled the air like the smell of earth after rain. The political excitement was personal and infectious and joyous. In the meantime, there were logistics. Most South Africans had never voted before. A large percentage of the population was illiterate and had to be educated. Because of the intimidation between supporters of Inkata, the Zulu party and the ANC, voter literacy was essential for the election to be 'free and fair'. People needed to understand that no-one could force them to vote for a particular party. The slogan of that era became 'Your vote is your secret'.

In the lead-up to the election, the fervour mounted, rolling like a storm towards a parched land. We kept lookout: the clouds are gathering, there will be rain. The revolution of coming rain. We all hoped for change, big and small: the end of sanctions and boycotts; a better economy; more jobs, less crime; housing and medical care for the poor; no more hunger; HIV treatment. South Africa would play and host international sports. No longer would foreigners spit at you when you said you were from South Africa. Tracy Chapman and Bruce Springsteen would visit. It was a time of reaching for the blue sky.

I returned to South Africa with teaching obligations to the Fulbright committee, so for the next two years I lectured in law at the University of the Witwatersrand, my alma mater. Though I fed off the energy and testosterone of young inquisitive men with progressive politics, and adored the smart bespectacled women who sat upfront and asked me impossible questions, academia was not for me. I'd spent a year at Yale 'thinking' about justice, and it was time to get my hands dirty. Also, the truth was that I didn't care enough about 'research' and 'publication'. Not in the way that mattered in academia.

The parting words of my lover at Yale (who had the annoying habit of referring to himself in the third person) were, 'Go back to South Africa, find the biggest mess you can and dive in head-first.' He could have said 'I love you'. But he was a Marxist and didn't understand the revolutionary power of love.

Back in South Africa, the Nationalist government had recently passed the Prevention of Family Violence Act, which legally acknowledged domestic violence for the first time. Though it was blunt and feeble, the first of its kind is groundbreaking in its own way by simply tendering a language, starting the conversation. From an advocacy point of view, even just a little something is better than a lot of nothing. I called WAGE and offered to train its counsellors on how to use this law. That phone-call marked the beginning of a long stretch of my life which took me into the pits of hell of the lives of so many South African women.

But I felt useful and inspired, a warrior in the fight to fix a broken but beautiful country. At last my big thighs seemed suitable for the task ahead.

Waking early on 27 April 1994 to a perfect Highveld spring day, I raced to switch on the TV. In front of me, Penny (pink and blonde) and Thabo (brown and suave) bubbled animatedly: 'And now we switch to Alexandra where the crowd has formed a long queue outside Alexandra High School.' An endless human-headed centipede snaked, patient as the earth, ID books in hand, some in Sunday best, others in work overalls, some dressed in African cloths and blankets, as the line in front of them promised a full day in the sun for the long-awaited right to place an X in a box.

The day before, a friend's mother told us she'd been shopping in an expensive clothes store when a black man in paint-stained work overalls came in, clutching what must have been several months' worth of wages in his hands, to buy a suit. 'To wear when I go to vote,' he announced.

Violet led the way, accompanying me, my parents and sisters to vote, she for the first time. I wore a t-shirt I'd picked up in a flea market in Manhattan, 'Love See No Colour'. In the streets we sang '*Shosholoza*', '*Nkosi Sikelel' iAfrica*' and we toyi-toyied, an African rhythmic dance. A boom-box appeared from somewhere playing African music.

There's no way to describe this moment without lapsing into the worst *schmaltzy* stereotypes. So let me just paint it for you: strangers hugged and held hands. People sang freedom songs. It was Woodstock, a Sunday gospel church service in the streets, Buddhist love in its most encompassing, undiscriminating and euphoric. Our common purpose felt spiritual, as if we could change universal karma, right the injustices of the past, and separate the good from the bad. The eyes of the world were on us as we stood in our long queues to cast our votes.

Hugging Violet, I chirped, 'Vi, isn't this wonderful?'

She shrugged, 'Ja, but nothing will change . . .'

'What do you mean?'

'Tomorrow, what will happen? Will I get a house? Will I get a car?' she huffed.

'Well maybe not tomorrow . . .' I blathered. 'But things will change slowly and they will become big changes . . . and . . .'

'We'll see,' she said, clicking her tongue and pushing me forward in the line as we edged closer to the voting booths.

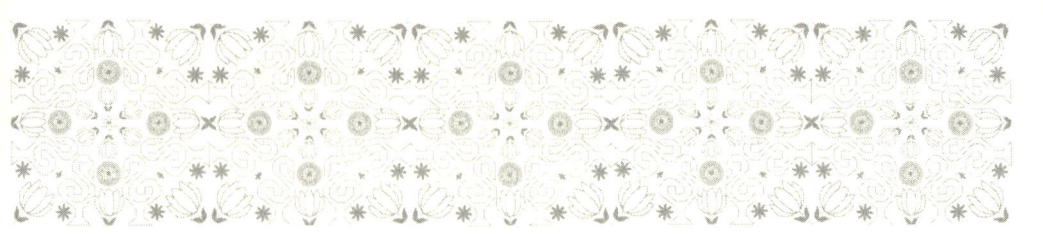

18
Small bites

*The best way to eat the elephant standing in your path
is to cut it up into little pieces.*
AFRICAN PROVERB

Something frightening has happened after two weeks on this eating plan. I've started tidying the apartment. It began with me sorting out the grocery cupboard while I was looking for low-fat rice crackers – you know, the ten I'm allowed to eat at morning tea? I find them right at the back of the cupboard and am suddenly beleaguered by the haphazard mixture of tins, biscuits, cereals and jars stuffed in there. I get the hell in and take everything out of the cupboard and begin neatly and systematically repacking it with the tins all on one shelf (the tuna tins stacked neatly one on top of the other), all the pasta in one large Tupperware container, and the bottles all on another shelf. I throw away everything that's out of date and mouldy.

I'm a hoarder. Why would that surprise me? There's no way on God's sweet earth that I'll ever starve, even if I tried very hard. I could feed all the guests at a huge *barmitzvah* with the contents of my cupboard. What's in there is a literal and rather embarrassing monument to the 'take-a-banana' principle.

Once I've got the kitchen cupboards under control, I move to the bathroom, throwing out ointments long past their expiry date, old caked soaps, half-used shampoos and those disgusting little shower caps I've collected from various holiday motels just in case there's ever a shortage of those. Do I have a collecting tic? Is this perhaps an accumulation disorder? Have I ever actually worn one of those shower caps in my entire life? Does *anybody* wear them?

Next I tackle the bedrooms, going through my wardrobes and getting rid of all old, daggy, shapeless, unfashionably unsalvageable clothing I hope I won't ever have so little self-esteem to wear again.

After filling a good few black garbage bags with my clothes for the charity bin, I zip through Jordan's room, sorting out his Pokemon, Yu-Gi-Oh! and football cards.

I find myself stopping short at the door to Shannon's room. I survey the carnage of stuffed toys, papers, Textas, bits of cloth she's making things from, saxophone music, dirty and clean clothes strewn everywhere, towels, iceblock wrappers, books and CDs. Her tribe of stuffed toys. This child cannot, will not, throw anything out. She keeps, collects and gathers everything. I simply can't imagine where she gets this from. Maybe it's a cry for help — an anxiety disorder she's inherited from having to leave South Africa and everything she loved behind. Maybe I over-identify, which is why I've never been strict enough to enforce any form of regimented disposal.

I know my limitations. I call Zed and implore him to help.

Despite my recent outburst, tidiness, much like skinniness, is not, in fact, my natural tendency. I am by nature *other things*. Chaotic. Creative. I'll concede even a little messy. Zed, by contrast, is both neat and a minimalist. As a marathon runner, he is organised and plans things. He needs nothing more than a water bottle strapped to his arm and a road and the man is happy as.

He stands at the doorway of Shannon's room for a moment then looks away, as one might from the carnage occasioned by a car crash. 'I can't,' he shrugs.

'What do you mean?' I cry.

'It's beyond my skills.'

'But this is your strength,' I hiss. 'You understand neat. Your genes are lined up in neat little rows, two by two. They're probably colour co-ordinated. Do *not* turn away.'

But he refuses, saying he's never had to tidy up such a big mess because he's never let things get to a point where they're this out of hand.

'Just start her off,' I stammer. 'You don't have to sort out the whole room, just point her in the right direction.'

But he's either unwilling or unable, which is his loss because sex is no longer a marital right but a privilege, a fact which in this moment seems to have slipped his tidy brain. He insists that neatness is a state of mind, not a quick fix. Apparently just putting all the books in the bookshelf isn't going to change a long-established system of squalor.

But I'm not asking him to change who Shannon is. I'm not even asking him to tidy her room. Shannon's not going to transform into an orderly individual who puts her dirty socks in the laundry and files all her schoolwork, even with his help.

Likewise, I'm not going to change my eating habits in a week. It's taken me nearly forty years to acquire my consumption patterns. Reversing them is a process that's going to call for patience, a long-term vision and stamina. I'm thinking *The*

Shawshank Redemption. One pocketful of sand every day. You wouldn't think it was much.

If a system needs to be changed you have to start somewhere. You can start with what's in front of you. You can start with what you can do. Small bites. In Shannon's case, one sock, one paper, one dirty towel at a time.

In my case, skim-milk cappuccinos from now on. No sugar in my tea or coffee. A cup of miso soup before tonight's meal, then again tomorrow, then again the next day. Brushing teeth straight after dinner (because nothing and I mean nothing tastes good after toothpaste). We're not talking the invasive conquests of stomach stapling, jaw-wiring or liposuction. I'm going with tiny changes which, over time, will add up. One cappuccino, one sip of soup at a time.

If you can tunnel your way out of jail with baby steps, you can tunnel your way out of obesity too.

I'll need to talk to Shannon about this problem. But I might have to get my own house in order first.

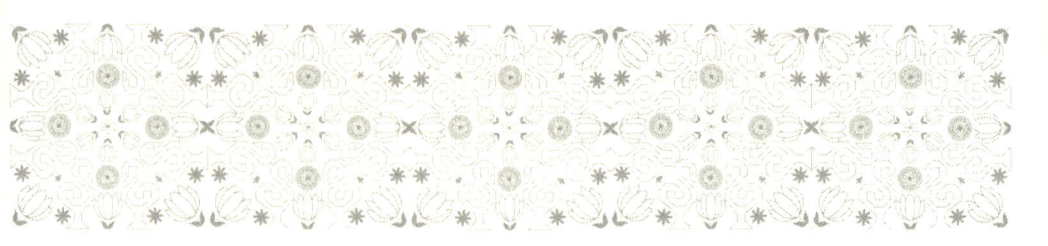

19
Coincidence #1

A child's tears reach the heavens.
YIDDISH PROVERB

Violet drank her tea with full-cream milk and four spoons of sugar from an enamel mug, the kind every South African domestic worker had, because an enamel mug couldn't shatter if dropped and so wouldn't need to be replaced. It's uncomfortable to drink tea from an enamel mug, because in addition to being unbreakable, enamel is also a very efficient conductor of heat. If there was no full-cream milk, Violet preferred her tea black rather than sullied with watery white man's skim milk, and would add an extra spoon or two of sugar over and above her usual four to compensate. When she sometimes let me sip her tea, my teeth would ache from the sweetness.

On Sundays, Violet would dress up for the Zion Christian Church service in one of the dazzling homemade outfits of vivid African cloth that she'd stitched on her sewing machine. Sometimes she even sported a little beret and a hand-me-down leather handbag of my mother's. In those moments,

COINCIDENCE #1

out of her pastel domestic worker's uniform, I glimpsed the matriarch in her, the woman who'd consciously chosen not to marry, who'd brought up two daughters on her own and who'd found resourceful ways of making extra money to send home. I don't think she was religious, and I doubt she believed in God. She was a pragmatist through and through and, if she thought men were too much trouble, chances are she had her reservations about the Almighty too. But church was one of the best places to tout for business for her *shebeen*.

Even though it was illegal, my folks didn't object to the home-brewed beer business she ran from our backyard so long as there was no trouble. On occasion, we'd hear her throwing drunken men out of her room with a lash of Sotho curses before they fled down our driveway. She was a strong woman, intolerant of nonsense, who didn't seem afraid of anything.

Unlike Violet, I've always been a bit of a frilly-blouse. I don't know how fear gets us – whether it's ingrained in the DNA, or seeps into us slowly like pickling spice. But as a child I was in and out of hospital after an accident with a broken bottle which tore the tendons in my left hand. I then developed a nauseating dread of hospitals and anyone whose smell reminded me of them, including doctors and various forms of detergent.

After that, fear, like a bullying older sibling who claims priority and insists on going first, sneaked its way into my relationships with all things. I was – and still am, terrified of roller-coasters, sharks, bluebottles, spiders, cold water, anesthetics, tidal waves, crowds, wasps, disfigurement, nuclear destruction and cancer, just to mention a few. Though it's probably normal to be afraid of these things, I was suffocated by my anxieties, causing me as a child to have recurring night terrors and ongoing headaches by day.

When I first got my head around the concept of death, I was genuinely appalled that God expected people to carry on as though it was just something unpleasant to be tolerated, like a dribbly old aunty who insists on hello and goodbye kisses. Through my childhood years, I barely held it together suppressing my horror at the thought that in one catastrophic moment the people you loved could be swept away by a tidal wave, struck down by a bolt of lightning, a galloping disease, a murderer's blade, a stray bullet or a speeding car. I often ran through in my mind the myriad ways there are to die and wondered variously whether I'd prefer to die by fire or water, by car accident or lingering disease, and decided none, thank you all the same. Yet there it was: death. Unavoidable and perfectly horrific.

Death seemed closer by night, that long lonely stretch where nightmares took advantage of the shadows. I always felt a sadness filter into me as the gloaming settled and I had to go upstairs to my bedroom, alone.

Many years later, I came across Virginia Woolf's unpublished writings, 'Moments of Being', in which she describes a childhood memory overhearing her parents talking about a man they knew who had committed suicide. Then walking in the garden one moonlit night, she saw an apple tree and inexplicably associated it with the horror of death.

I know this ability to make improbable but potent associations all too well. It may be a gift of a heightened imagination, but it burdens the psyche with irrational fears. I remember one particular night in my childhood when my parents were out, and I lay wide-eyed alone in my bed, an insomniac already at the age of eight. Violet knew how I hated the dark, so she'd often come and lie next to me until I fell asleep. But on this night she was downstairs as a thunderstorm broke, one

COINCIDENCE #1

of those violent cataclysms of lightning and thunder a small child struggles not to take personally. Suddenly the light in the passageway went out. I could hear Violet bumping around downstairs, scrabbling for a torch or match so she could make her way through the obstacle course in my father's studio to flick the trip switch back up. I held my breath but nothing happened.

Put the lights back on, Vi, put them on, I wished. Time seemed stuck. I tried not to think that rain made roads wet and slippery, or that Mom and Dad were driving in the rain, or that car accidents happened in the rain. '*Please, God, don't worry about the lights, just bring Mom and Dad home . . .*' I bargained. '*I don't care about the dark or the rain, just don't let there be an accident . . . bring them home safely . . . please, please . . . just bring them home . . .*' I whispered.

And right then I heard my parents' car throttling up our driveway.

Now, remember, I was only eight. I couldn't even *spell* coincidence. I still had expectations of the Tooth Fairy, for heaven's sake. And with the purity of that consciousness, I understood: I had asked God for something and gotten it.

Philosophers actually have a fancy name for this moment of illumination: a rapturous encounter. Apparently people pay good money in ashrams and monasteries to experience a moment of clarity such as this. It certainly got my attention and routed a synapse in my brain that I've never, despite frequent doubts to the contrary, quite been able to disengage – an eerie sense that God actually *listens*. That encounter in my bed in the rainy darkness was the genesis of the spiritual awakening I'd come to know many years later as the three-verbed mantra: ask, believe, receive.

This brings me to one of my favourite stories about my *zaide*, who was once castigated by a rabbi for talking in synagogue. 'Mr Fedler, please,' the rabbi said, 'We come to *shul* to pray.'

'Pray?' my *zaide* said incredulously. 'Pray I can do at home. I come to *shul* to talk to my friends.'

I've never much been one for synagogue. But I am in frequent conversation with God. He's a good listener who never interrupts.

And occasionally He acknowledges one's efforts.

20

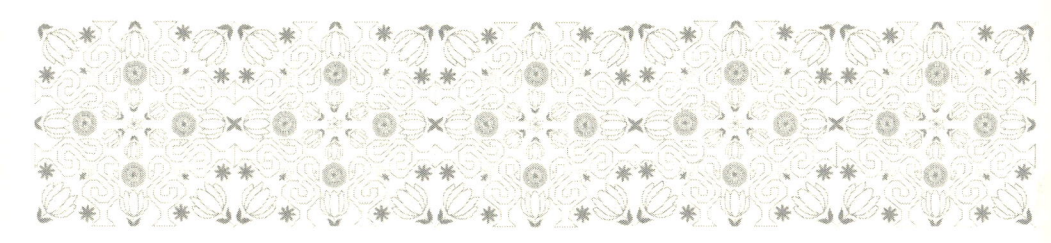

Run

You do not teach a giraffe to run.
SOTHO PROVERB

'God give me strength,' I mutter under my breath. I'm standing at the counter of my local coffee shop, Gusto, waiting on my large skinny cappuccino, no sugar. In front of me, encased in glass, is a row of mini cheesecakes dripping with passionfruit nectar, caramel kisses with chocolate topping and gingerbread pear cake. I avert my eyes and grab my coffee when it arrives, moving away from the array of delicacies offering me a million ways to be obese. Thank God coffee is allowed on my eating plan. In the past I've tried some of those malicious detox diets in which one must forgo coffee, alcohol, milk, wheat and anything that isn't a fruit or a vegetable, and unless I'm missing something, life's too short to be that miserable.

When it comes to sacrifice, you have to weigh up what you can and cannot live without. I'm not a big fan of the biblical story of God telling Abraham to sacrifice his son Isaac on the altar because I myself am not a prankster, and I certainly have no interest in a God with sadistic tendencies. I've dated a few men like that and, frankly, they weren't worth the effort and the sex was weird. I know God said, 'Only kidding – a ram will do,' at the crucial moment. But as a mother, I worry that Isaac would never again have been able to completely relax whenever he saw his old man reach for a knife to carve the Sabbath roast.

Cutting out seconds, *schmaltz* and fries is not, admittedly, in the same camp as being asked to slaughter one's only child for whom one has waited ninety-nine years, but both of them sit firmly on the 'Not-Much-Fun' side of the fence. Losing weight is a moment-by-moment sacrifice, ongoing suffering and discomfort propelled by the larger forces of vanity and the desire to live longer.

The Buddhists have really nailed us on this one: we are indeed suffering-averse, pleasure-seeking physical beings. Buddhism suggests that we should a) acknowledge that we are suffering-averse, pleasure-seeking physical beings – in other words, not be in denial – and b) become okay with this rather spiritually diminutive condition of ours by not beating ourselves up every time we think about a chicken burrito with or without the jalapeños rather than concentrating on the white light on the in-breath and the blue light on the out-breath.

Given that these are lifelong pursuits calling for impressive spiritual discipline, meditation, introspection and insight into what a single hand clapping sounds like, the best one can strive for when it comes to losing weight is: this is gonna hurt but I'm not gonna cry. Just like Abraham who followed God's instruction, we have to go through the motions and hope at some point for redemption from our suffering.

Nowhere is this more apparent than when it comes to the question of exercise, the benefits of which, the experts claim, range from preventing cancer to improving your sex life, managing your weight, improving your sleep, and strengthening your heart and lungs.

My father, badgered by all the health propaganda about living longer and increasing mobility, joined a gym in the past few years. Whenever I ask him how it's going, he sighs, 'Oy, don't ask. Why does it have to be such an effort? I've got a Jewish body. It likes to sit in a chair.' Mercifully for him, gyms have bikes for Jewish bodies in which you can sit while pedalling. There are also rowing machines for the Semitic temperament where you can work out while prone.

The Jewish contribution to world affairs (politics, medicine, psychology, entertainment, literature, science and medicine) is inversely proportional to its sporting achievements, unless chess can be considered a sport, and I think a line has to be drawn somewhere. Exercise, it seems, is not very Jewish. The Jews may have crossed the desert, but it would've been more an amble than a power walk – it took us forty *years.*

Jews, however, have a reputation for excelling at maths, though that basket of genes didn't find its way through the DNA forests to my little cottage. I understand the rudiments of addition and subtraction (I get the notions of 'more' and 'less', especially when it comes to chocolate mousse) but parabolas, sine, cos and tan functions make my temples ache. I've never understood what these squiggles of gibberish signify, no matter how many times my teachers tried explaining them to me.

Unfortunately, there are two mathematical components to this weight loss curriculum. On the food side, I have to decrease my activity. On the exercise side, I have to increase my activity. Less fuel. More action. The action burns the fuel, and I lose weight.

Apparently, to lose one kilogram I have to burn 32,000 kilojoules. If I cut 1000 kilojoules from my daily diet, I could lose that kilogram in about a month. If I added thirty minutes of brisk walking to my daily routine, I could burn another 600 kilojoules a day. If I increase that to an hour of brisk walking, as opposed to the meandering window-shopping pace I am comfortable with, I could burn another 1200 kilojoules a day.

This does prompt the question: what's a kilojoule? I'm glad you asked. I have no idea. I have read numerous definitions which say 'a unit of energy', but I still don't get it. I just know that food has them and you need to consume less of them if you want to get skinny.

Despite my ancestral deficiency in sports, I start exercising with a vengeance. The problem is that the heavier you are, the more of you has to move for it to qualify as exercise.

In my early twenties (when I was, believe it or not, a qualified aerobics instructor) I could do a hundred high kicks – the kind where your knee touches your nose – to the sound of Paddy Hines's 'Chain Gang'. I was once scarily fit, long before stretchmarks, when it mattered whether I waxed my legs or not. But that was then.

Right now, when it comes to exercise, my goal is to keep it up for as long as I can without vomiting or injuring myself, which is ominously possible when almost a hundred kilos of flesh is moving through space at a rapid speed on a temperamental spine.

So I begin on Coogee oval with a simple three-letter word: R-U-N. But it's as if my brain has just taken up Cantonese and my muscles are all Bulgarian.

Brain: 'Okay, run, Joanne, run . . .'

Legs: 'You want me to do what?'

Brain: 'Run.'

Legs: 'What do you mean?'

Brain: 'Run . . . you know . . . Like walking, but more quickly.'

Legs: 'Like this?'

Brain: 'No, faster . . .'

Legs: 'Like this?'

Brain: 'What's the matter with you? RUN!'

When I get my legs to do something that I think approximates running, I tell myself that if I can just keep it up for one whole minute, that will be a spectacular achievement. Tomorrow I will improve on it 100 per cent by running for two whole minutes. Bite-size chunks. One step at a time.

Let's leave me running around Coogee oval for a moment while I tell you the story of Laura Schultz, a sixty-three-year-old grandmother in the United States who, by all accounts, lifted up the back end of a Buick to get it off her grandson's arm. When interviewed about the incident, she said she didn't want to talk about it. When she finally did talk about it, she said it was uncomfortable for her to think about what she had done because it challenged her beliefs about what is possible . . . and left her wondering: 'What does it say about the rest of my life? Have I wasted it?'

Okay, back to me running and here's my point: I run for *seventeen minutes* without stopping. I mean, my limbs are all still intact and I can breathe, sort of.

WHEN HUNGRY, EAT

In this moment, I love my body. I love what it can do.
This thing I say a lot: 'I can't...' I wonder about it. I really do.

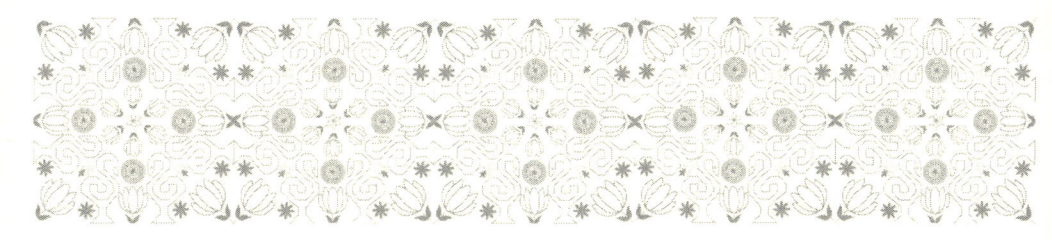

21
Consumption

If nothing is going well, call your grandmother.
ITALIAN PROVERB

No matter how hard I try, I simply can't imagine my Granny Bee, who was a little sparrow of a woman, lifting a Buick to get it off my arm. Though, being an incorrigible flirt, she'd probably have been able to charm a dozen passers-by into helping.

'Your pa saved my life,' she once told me.

This wasn't the sort of thing I expected her to say about my grandfather. She and my grandfather had been unhappily married, and she'd spent her life in love with another man. I'd just asked her if she was sorry she'd never married her true love, and that's when she said, 'No ... no, my darling. If I hadn't married your pa, I would have died when I was a young woman, well before your mother was born. Your pa saved my life.'

Since my father's mother, *Bobba* Chaya, had died when he was just thirteen, Granny Bee, my mother's mother, was the only granny I knew. She was breathtakingly beautiful (I'm talking film-star looks), formally uneducated, every inch a lady, skinny in the waist with a huge bosom and still stylish in stilettos into her eighties. As I grew out of being her little Jo, I towered over her, at a few inches short of six foot. I think I bewildered her. I was certainly not what girls were supposed to grow into. She loved me utterly, inexplicably; even when I turned into a woman she didn't begin to understand – an outspoken feminist. An activist. Did those words have any meaning to her?

During my years at WAGE I stopped shaving under my arms, a glimpse of which would cause her to clutch her chest and exhale, 'Oh my God,' though she elegantly restrained herself from saying anything more. She also choked back her shock when I fell in love with a black man who was, in her English upbringing, a 'Bantu'. She used to gaily recite the poem, '*My little golly is black as ink, not like my dolly, nice and pink*'. I once told her it was racist. She said, 'I don't see why – golliwogs *are* black, after all . . .' And that was the end of that.

When I fell pregnant out of wedlock with Zed's child, making social introductions rather awkward, she made no fuss, certainly not to my face, though she often mentioned what a 'lovely fellow' Zed was – 'Indeed, the kind of nice, ordinary bloke one ought to settle down with.'

Being a lovely fellow, however, wasn't the measure by which she judged men. Neither was wealth. Kindness and generosity were well and good, but not a clincher. No, a man simply had to be handsome. 'When it comes to marriage, be practical, my darling,' she once told me in hushed tones. 'Remember, you have to look at him for a very long time.' She never tired of a good-looking man and was still watching Wimbledon assiduously until her very last days for that 'gorgeous Agassi'.

CONSUMPTION

My fine-looking grandfather Jack had pursued her shamelessly, after catching a glimpse of her at just seventeen. She told me he'd seen her standing on a balcony as he was driving past and turned to his two passengers, announcing, 'You see that little girl up there? That's the girl I'm going to marry.' I've always considered claims of 'love at first sight' ridiculous. Measuring love (that slow, deep, abiding emotion) by a swift rush of endorphins to the groin, if indeed endorphins even go south, seems the height of idiocy and I don't like to attribute such unflattering qualities to my beloved pa. Nonetheless, Jack 'fell in love' with my granny with just one look, and two years later he had convinced her to marry him, though she was – and would, it turns out, always be – in love with her childhood sweetheart, David. David was given the chance to snatch her back, but he 'wasn't ready', and urged my granny to wait for him. But she didn't – a choice that caused her, David and my grandfather much heartache over many years.

On the fourth day of her honeymoon in London, my granny began to cough uncontrollably, bringing up blood. Within hours she was admitted to hospital where x-rays were taken and she was diagnosed with tuberculosis. The doctors told her that she was incredibly lucky that she'd come to England on honeymoon and caught a chill that had revealed the consumption. It was nothing short of a divine coincidence.

She told me how my pa Jack cared for her during the six weeks she spent in hospital recuperating and how she became his muse – after their abortive honeymoon, Jack, who was already a qualified lawyer, returned to university and became a doctor. Medicine had always been his primary passion but his own father had talked him out of it, no doubt having had a bad experience at some point in time with a person in a white coat.

Had my granny held his advances at bay and waited for David, within a few years the galloping consumption would have affected both her lungs and by then it would have been too late. And so, it was David's fear of commitment that both broke her heart and saved her life.

When she finally fell pregnant after eight years of trying, the Second World War had just broken out. Though she agonised about whether it was right or safe to bring a child into this world, she never regretted having my mother. In her eyes, she was her 'angel', 'the perfect daughter who never gave her a moment's worry or trouble'. Unlike my sisters and I, she often reminded me. We, apparently, were unrelentingly troublesome and didn't give my mother a minute's respite from anxiety.

After many years of trying for a second baby, she miscarried in the fifth month of pregnancy ('I believe it was a boy') and of this loss, she simply said, 'At the time it worries you, but you just get over it.'

'Just getting over it' was her philosophy in life, capturing the Victorian repression of all emotion she was taught to adopt. Tragedy had struck when she was sixteen, with the death of her mother, Doris, from tuberculosis at just thirty-six, and, in her own moving words, 'The world fell to pieces'. This description is the closest I ever came to knowing anything about her feelings. She was left alone to process her mother's death, forced to hold her grief with ladylike composure.

Granny Bee wasn't a religious woman. I don't think she believed in God, though she probably had a soft spot for Jesus, with that lovely beard and all, despite being Jewish. She was anxious and nervous and deeply terrified of a long, lingering death. But she was gracious and a wonderful hostess and believed that two occasions should never be passed up: the opportunity to utter a kind word and to have a whiskey on ice, which she did every day at four pm sharp, with the words, *'Op ons'* – Afrikaans for 'On us', not 'Up yours'.

Some years before she died, Granny Bee handed me a little golden locket containing two ancient sepia photos. 'Elizabeth and Solomon Solomon, my mother's grandparents. They're buried in an old cemetery in Melbourne. I want you to have this,' she said, pressing it into my palm.

'Melbourne? As in Australia?' I asked. 'What were they doing there?'

And that's when I first discovered that her mother, Doris, had been born in Australia. Doris's grandparents migrated from England on the SS *Calcutta* in 1854 when Solomon landed a contract to build a railway bridge across Melbourne's Yarra River. It took them seventy-two days to reach Australian soil on an 1800-tonne steamship full of livestock, with a handful of human passengers, Elizabeth being the only woman. Her daughter Hannah married Myer Myers, who had come to Australia from Birmingham during the gold rush. He hadn't had much success in Ballarat, so when gold was discovered in South Africa at the turn of the century, he uprooted his family and followed the crowd to Africa.

A decade later, I would take my family from the bosom of Africa and backtrack to the Antipodes to start a new life, with that little locket somewhere in my possessions.

22

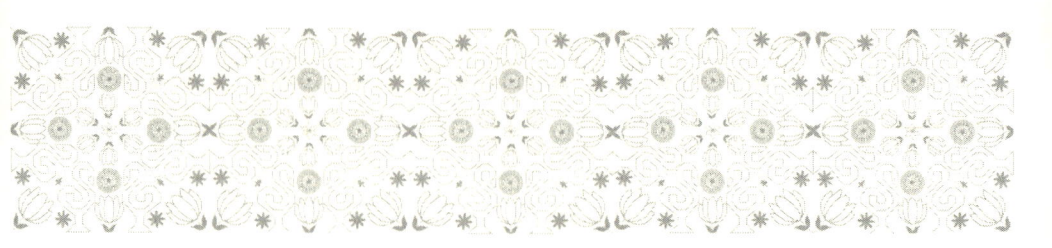

Crisp

A fly does not mind drowning in coconut cream.
SWAHILI PROVERB

Shannon and Jordan are fighting over the *latkes*. They both want to help me fry them. But a frying pan full of scalding oil and two under-tens bickering around the stove with egglifters in their hands do not make for a relaxing afternoon. I might have to take a preventative headache tablet.

Okay, you're wondering why I'm deep-frying at this point in my life. And I really can pass this buck this time. It's because of Judas Maccabeus who led a Jewish uprising against the oppressive reign of King Antiochus and the Hellenists in 165 BC. When he and his men returned victorious to Jerusalem, they discovered the Temple had been desecrated and all but one of the oil lamps had been polluted. There was only enough olive oil to keep the lamp burning for a day, yet it burned miraculously for eight. And so in December, over a period of eight days, Jews celebrate the Festival of Lights with foods that have been fried in oil.

Judaism expresses its practice through victuals, and poetically too. The Passover plate with its shank bone, burned egg, salt water and bitter herbs all tell a story of sacrifice, tears and anguish. We eat *matza* because our ancestors didn't have time to wait for the bread to rise in Egypt before setting off. On *Rosh Hashana* (Jewish New Year), the table is laden with round, whole, complete foods (eggs, bagels, a round sweet bread filled with raisins) and one is just about obligated to eat such no-no's on the Food Fascist's list as honey cake and a mountain of chocolate to ensure a sweet new year.

Trying to instil peace between my offspring is therefore only the beginning of my problems, because the Festival of Lights, beginning tonight, should more accurately be called the Festival of *Schmaltz*. The miracle of the lamp will have nothing on the miracle I'm hoping for if the scales show a loss at the end of this week.

Maybe God doesn't want Jews to be skinny. What other faith forces a person to the deep-fryer with instructions to eat crispy golden *latkes*, the Jewish version of a hash brown, laden with cinnamon sugar? The problem is, I have the same resistance as an alcoholic at a wine-tasting when it comes to crispy things. This habit was instilled in me as a child while I sat at Granny Bee's table where crispiness was next to godliness.

Though she didn't look like a marvellous chef – I always imagined them to be large and ruddy – she effortlessly turned out gastronomic triumphs like roast beef with mustard sauce, crème caramels with caramelised sugar, and pickled fish smothered in circles of onion rings from her kitchen, around which she pottered in her high heels. Even an ordinary green salad was a sensation (her secret was to rub raw garlic onto the wooden salad-bowl which infused the leaves).

Eating at her table was a mélange of delights. Tap water became saffron, emerald and ruby jewels in their coloured bulbs of glass. Her silver mustard dishes with little blue glass holders and tiny silver spoons made even the dullest of hot dogs magical. Her specialty was duck with pineapple and ginger, which she cooked long and slow over a whole day to gently coax the thick subcutaneous fat out, which she then spooned back over the bird to create the fowl equivalent of pork crackling. She was the Queen of Crispy: roast potatoes in butter, butternut pumpkin caramelised in honey, the fatty bits on the lamb chops, the cheesy edges around the lasagne ... Good grief, I think I'm salivating.

When I was a child, everyone fought over the crispy chicken drumsticks and the wings. We had to take *turns* eating the parson's nose. The breast was left over for the loser who didn't get to stake their claim early enough – my dad, most likely, who'd sigh and accept his dry white-meat fate. So if I have any choice in the matter, I go for the wings. The crunchy bits. The bones. But these days I'm only allowed 'skinless chicken breast', which has no crispy bits to speak of. And crispy, let's face it, is where the party is.

In a perfect world, with no kilojoule karma, I'd live on a diet of deep-fried soft-shell crab, samoosas, anything tempura, agedashi tofu, doughnuts, spring rolls, prawn parcels and chicken wings. Lipids are the life of flavour and, to make matters worse, eating crispy things further stimulates our appetite through sound and texture. This is why it's almost impossible to stop after just one chip. But let's be adults here: crispy is nothing other than crunchy *schmaltz*. Every bite is another step towards a coronary. There are even gloomy intimations of crispy's alliance with cancer.

But Granny Bee didn't know or didn't care. In one meal, she could use the same quantity of butter a person, by the Food Fascist's standards, is allowed over a *year*. What's more, she retained her hourglass figure all the way into her geriatric years. She lived till the age of eighty-nine without any cancer, without joining a gym and, as far as I know, without ever going on a diet of any sort.

I remember her darting around the table in her high heels, dishing up seconds – 'Have a little more, my darling' – and only intermittently sitting to pick at the morsel on her plate. Come to think of it, while we were all putting on calories, she was working them off, flitting and dancing between the hotplate and our plates, but not lunging, as far as I can recall. I think she'd have found that vulgar. I remember her giving up the one little wing on her plate when someone else (probably me) wanted it as thirds, protesting how full she was from having spent all day in the kitchen tasting everything while she cooked.

People said, 'Bee, you eat like a bird.'

'Yes, like a vulture,' she'd giggle, though it was patently false and she knew it. Only skinny people can make those sorts of jokes.

Like French women, she ate whatever she liked. Crispy, *schmaltz*y, fatty. But she ate, as she did everything else, including drinking, smoking and flirting with every man, in seemingly effortless moderation. A trait I lamentably never inherited genetically nor imbibed sitting around her table.

We finally finish making the *latkes* which are all laid out on paper towel soaking up excess oil. I put six into a takeaway container.

'Who are those for?' Jordan asks.

'For Miriam. Will you take them over for me?'

There are a few grumbles, but the kids oblige. After all, tonight is the first of eight nights of *Chanukah* presents and no-one wants to jeopardise those. I tell you, all a mother needs is decent ammunition.

After an argument about who gets to hold the *latkes*, Shannon and Jordan set off together to ring on her bell. I remind them to 'be patient' as Miriam doesn't always hear it the first time. Miriam, I suppose doesn't expect many visitors. She has a single daughter who never married and is now too old to have children. As she told me this, she'd faltered. 'This is my greatest pain,' she'd confessed. 'Worse than the arthritis. You know, to have survived the Holocaust, but not to have any grandchildren ... ach ...' she'd sighed.

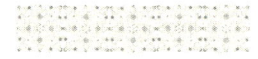

Tonight, after Shannon and Jordan have fought over who gets to light the *Chanukah* candles, I feel myself sinking into sadness that my little niece Jenna isn't here to share our *latkes* and sing songs with us. It's a lonely Festival of Lights without family. But I catch that thought before it slides into melancholy and instead I think of little Miriam, who is shrinking. And of her hunger for the grandchildren she'll never have.

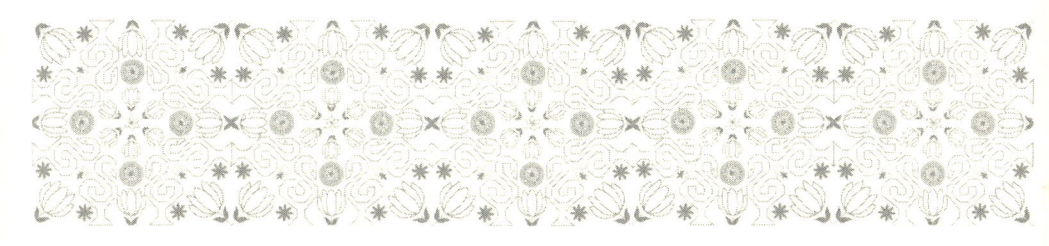

23
A ghastly poetry

*Be careful if you make a woman cry, because God
counts her tears.
A woman came out of a man's rib –
not from his feet to be walked on,
not from his head to be superior,
but from his side to be equal,
under the arm to be protected
and next to his heart to be loved.*
THE TALMUD

The essence of a healthy lifestyle is easy enough to remember: *everything in moderation*. My granny lived by that motto. But there are some things that are best avoided on one's plate, as well as in one's life. Murder, for example.

Even though I laughed as loudly as the next person watching John Travolta and Samuel L Jackson frantically mopping up brains and blood before the missus came home, in real life murder is nothing like a Tarantino film. I say this having once found myself at WAGE sitting at my desk opposite a woman whose sister had been stabbed to death by her boyfriend with a pair of scissors. Honest to God. A pair of 'please-pass-them-I-need-to-cut-this-label-off' scissors. I remember how icy cold my fingers became and how my saliva pooled under my tongue making it hard to swallow.

I had nothing to give this grieving woman other than a cup of tea and a shortbread biscuit, if they hadn't already all been snatched up. I don't recall what I said to her, other than the standard assurances that we would 'follow up' the case with the investigating officer. The verbal consolations and plans of action I tendered were crudely indistinguishable from one another, like an oncologist who develops a stock repertoire of phrases in breaking bad news over and over again.

My shock was mottled with that abysmal human affliction, morbid curiosity, the macabre magnetism that draws your eyes to the scene of a car crash though you know you don't want to see what's there. This poor woman had just returned from the mortuary after 'identifying the body'. I took in the facts of the fatal stabbing: the description of the corpse curled up like a foetus, her hands covering her face. How people articulate unspeakable things eludes me, but the words that find their way through grief have an adhesive quality becoming a ghastly poetry it's impossible to loosen from memory.

There was nothing comic about this. It was ordinary and bureaucratic and I wanted her to leave because the waiting room was full of people who hadn't yet been killed.

That day, with murder so close I could reach out and touch it, I slammed up against the concrete insight that I was on the wrong side of the problem. Women only came to see us *after* they'd been raped or battered or their sisters had been murdered. We needed to get to them *before* the violence did. Their lives were embedded in a complex chain of interlocking systems of poverty, racism and misogyny. These were *structures* of subjugation, not individual bad marriages or unlucky choices you could shrug off. Superman, you'll notice, only ever saved individuals. He never ended slavery, sexism or racism, which would have required him to rejig an entire system of oppression.

That day, I finally 'got' the inadequacies of the liberal human rights' view. In a society warped by its history, the problems people face cannot be cured like Seasonal Affective Disorder or a winter flu. They are systemic, congenital. Even with a good law on your side, AVOs still had to be enforced by police officers – the same police officers I'd overheard make remarks like, 'Women ask for it' and 'It's part of their (black) culture to hit, you know ...' AVOs couldn't address the real problems abused women face – they couldn't put food on the table or cover a sick child's antibiotics. They couldn't stop a man from drinking his salary away on a Friday night and returning home with beer on his breath and a fight in his fist. And often the *last* thing a battered woman wants is for her husband to go to jail if he provides the family's only source of income.

More and more, my work began to feel like being jabbed with the syringe of impotent rage day in and day out. My impatience didn't help. People who dither irritate me. Battered women are wafer-thin on self-worth and are not (how could they be?) capable decision-makers. I've got no tolerance for bullies, but what I shockingly discovered is that I get equally frustrated with people who don't take measures to protect themselves (and, even more maddeningly, their children).

I liked to think I was adding value to the world, but if I'm honest, I often lost my way. An old black woman once stood up at a meeting and addressed us as 'you white women who think rape is the worst thing that can happen'. We stared down at our folded hands in our laps, silenced by the blaze in her voice that came from an anguish we'd never visited, not even in our nightmares. In a tone that betrayed no indulgence or self-pity, she said, 'I was raped, my mother was raped, my grandmother was raped and my daughter was raped, and her children will be too. Stop telling us this is the worst thing that can happen to a woman. Tell the government we want housing, running water, health care. You can get used to rape. Living without those things is worse than rape.'

Compassion fatigue brings down more than just the walls of our idealism. It kicks the feet out from our ability to look strangers in the eye and our willingness to be kind to another person. It's a form of emotional collapse, and I was falling. Too much ugliness leaches your dreams out of you. Stories dropped from their thread, like beads off a broken necklace.

Many years later, I'd return to the site of the slow torture of my spirit. I'd find the place where the belly of my heart had been slit open, causing its contents to leak like a torn bag of rice until it was emptied. Only then would I understand that the human psyche isn't an alimentary canal, but a spider's web. Whatever goes in becomes entangled in the sinew, the muscle, the bone of the spirit. We hold everything unless we consciously let it go.

It took years. A slow dawning realisation that I wasn't feeding a hunger. I was starving alongside my clients.

I left WAGE brittle, hoping like hell to forget every single one of those women.

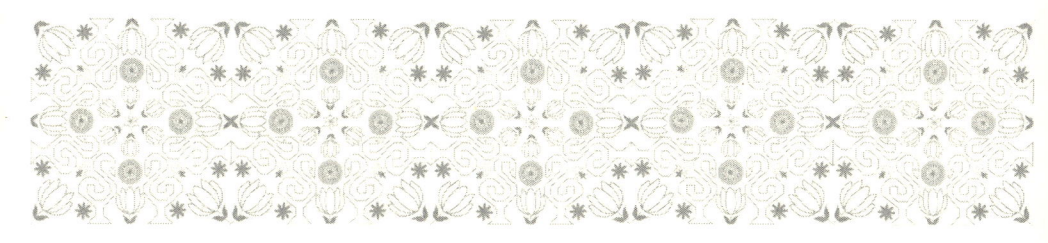

24
Burp

The best memory is that which forgets nothing but injuries.
Write kindness in marble and write injuries in the dust.
IRANIAN PROVERB

I've put a photograph of myself up on the fridge. It's not a flattering picture. In one hand I'm holding a large bone, the remains of a leg of lamb I've just finished gnawing clean. In the other is a beer bottle. It's the kind of photograph you'd probably not put up on a dating website were you, say, trying to attract members of the opposite sex. Zed took this shot because my fondness for eating the bones is a source of much mirth in the conservatory of his humour. He used it on a birthday card once, with something like 'You're so sexy with a bone in your hand' scribbled beneath it. He's clever with words like that.

This gluttonous, flabby, beer-swilling profile is on the fridge as a reminder: this is not who I want to be. And that angle makes my nose look even bigger than it is in real life.

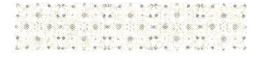

'In real life' is the phrase Jordan uses when seeking reassurance about the non-existence of ghosts, aliens or Dementors (thanks, JK, thanks a lot). 'There's no such thing in *real* life is there, Mum?' Real life being where imagination can't get you.

The other day he grumbled in from school, thumped his schoolbag against the wall when I asked him to do his homework and called Shannon a moron for getting to the toilet before him. After I'd yelled, imposed a TV and Nintendo DS ban, fed him two-minute noodles just in case his blood sugar was low, poor little brat, and confiscated the broom he was using to clout the pot plant, it finally came out: 'Rufus Kremansky said my mum looks like a witch.'

I suppressed the urge to encourage him to pee in Rufus Kremansky's lunch box or to tease him about his silly name. I am, after all, an adult.

'Don't let it upset you,' I consoled. 'I do have a big nose.'

'Yes, but you don't look like a witch!' he mumbled.

'Well, maybe a good witch . . .' I suggested. 'You know, like Nanny McPhee.'

'But there's no such thing in real life,' he quipped.

It really is my cross to bear, if I may be excused for mixing religious metaphors, that I have an unmistakably Jewish nose. Mine is the stereotypically large facial protuberance depicted in anti-Semitic jokes and cartoons. The joke in our family goes that if you place me and my cousin Alan, who also has a massive konk, back to back, you have a pick-axe. Plastic surgeons have been known, upon beholding my profile, to get a certain glint in their eyes.

Despite the lures of cosmetic rhinoplasties and the cruelties of playground banter, I have stuck with the nose God gave me. Apart from how little the prospect of having my facial bones broken appeals to me, I've never found my nose as offensive as others have. This nose has travelled a long way through Jewish history to end up on my face. And I think one has to respect the tenacity of genetic perseverance.

My nose reminds me of who I am, and equally who I will never be; that is, Demi Moore or Angelina Jolie. It holds me close to my history, like my photograph albums, the videos of the kids when they were little, the handwritten letters of lovers past, the curls from Shannon and Jordan's first haircuts, their lost teeth and every certificate I've kept in treasure boxes at the top of my cupboard. Come to think of it, my small problem with nostalgia could turn out to be more a dilemma of storage.

In Yiddish there's a saying: 'No-one but a fool trips on what's behind him.' It's such a sensible reminder to stop looking back and to concentrate on what's in front of you. Lot's poor wife certainly learned that lesson the hard way when she was turned into a pillar of salt. A poem which has haunted me since my days of studying English literature is Tennyson's 'Mariana', equally beautiful and suicidally depressing:

> *Old faces glimmer'd thro the doors,*
> *Old footsteps trod the upper floors,*
> *Old voices called her from without.*
> *She only said, 'My life is dreary,*
> *He cometh not,' she said,*
> *She said, 'I am aweary, aweary,*
> *I would that I were dead!'*

I can't quite make my mind up about remembering – is it good for us, like bran, or bad for us, like mixing drinks? I love to remember all the thrilling and joyous moments in my life, but since they've passed and I'm now living an unthrilling domestic existence, that's sort of sad. Whenever I watch old footage of when the kids were babies or flick through the photo albums of my youth, I always feel an emptiness at the end. My kids are getting bigger and cheekier by the hour. Recall always makes me feel what I've lost. It's a clue that too much remembering can easily become a sickness of the spirit and go the 'Mariana' way.

But there are other ways to remember.

My friend Jane is a photo-displayer and has dozens of photos of her two gorgeous kids, Chad and Kaitlyn, on her fridge, on the walls, on the dresser and on a corkboard in the kitchen. Two of the photos are difficult to look at. They're of Kaitlyn lying in a tiny hospital bed with pipes coming out of her little body, like a chicken with tentacles. Kaitlyn was born with Stickler syndrome and, as well as the congenital defects, she has fought for her life on a few occasions. I once asked Jane why she keeps these photos up. 'Don't they freak you out?'

'No,' she replied, 'they remind me that she's still here.'

Remembering in this way is an act of gratitude.

To Jews, the act of remembrance is both sacred and compulsory. In prayer services, four times a year there's a special memorial portion, *Yizkor*, devoted to remembering the dead. The Jewish groom breaks a glass under the *chuppah* (wedding canopy) to recall the destruction of the Temple, reminding the bridal couple and all their friends and family that 'Despite this deliriously happy moment, oy, have we suffered in the past!' Jews have an idiomatic convention of speaking about historical events as if they happened to us personally: *we* were slaves in Egypt (not just our ancestors); *we* were on trains to Auschwitz (not just our forefathers). This, I've heard it explained, is a prompt to stay connected to human suffering even after the pain has passed. En masse, as part of a tribal identity, this 'When–We' custom is called 'commemoration'.

BURP

Don't get me wrong – I'm all for a good commemoration to honour past suffering and display appreciation for the fact that it's over. But Jews can overindulge in remembering, as if memory itself were a *barmitzvah* buffet of smoked salmon bagels. By Jewish standards, remembering could probably qualify as a profession.

Buddhists are less hung up on remembrance. Dwelling on the past, much like dreaming about the future, absents us from this moment, the only place that's real and in which it's possible to change how we feel, think and act. It's the single location of choice; the womb of karma. My Buddhist teacher Thanissara says, 'Wanting what is not here stops us from being here.'

Hillel, in 'Ethics of the Fathers', expresses a similar call to be present in the moment: 'If am not for myself, who will be for me? If I am only for myself, what am I? And if not now, when?'

Like peristalsis and breathing, remembering is instinctive. It may be impossible to stop ourselves from going there, just as trying to suppress a burp will lead to indigestion (and what is a burp if not a memory of lunch gone by?). Memories find their way in, whether they have to sneak in through the back door of our dreams, or tunnel underground through our subconscious. But what if we're not complete prey to the hungers of memory? What if we could wean ourselves from too much of it? Maybe we can make healthier, more conscious memory choices so we don't linger in places that fatten us with incurable sorrows and vanished happiness.

I look long and hard at the picture on the fridge.

I need to find a better picture.

One that doesn't feel like a wound.

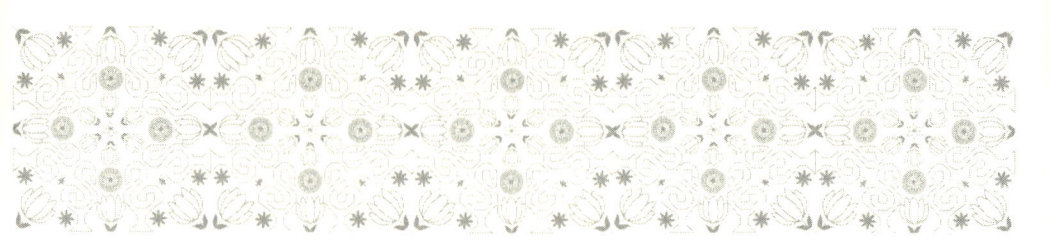

25
Coincidence #2

God sends the weather according to your needs.
Yiddish proverb

My father became very religious when I was about ten years old. It seemed to happen overnight, the way a nasty virus might nab you. It was as if someone had cast a *Lubavitch* spell on him or put him under *Chassidic* hypnosis. Three days without a shave and suddenly he had a beard, wore a black hat and invoked a tonne of rules, 613 to be exact, which set out when to say a prayer, refrain from eating this or that, light candles, and say amen. He roped our whole family into whatever pact he'd made with God, and as a result our entire house was koshered (separate eating utensils for meat and milk) in a protracted ritual with a pentacle of rabbis in which cutlery was buried in the ground and blessings recited over crockery. My dad then prayed every morning decked out in phylacteries and piously attended synagogue on Saturdays and lectures on a Thursday night where, I am led to believe, a great deal of herring and whiskey was consumed.

COINCIDENCE #2

As the indirect beneficiary of his new-found faith, I was sent to a rabbi every Sunday morning to learn how to become a good Jewish girl. Under this rabbi's tutelage, I learned the rules of *kashrut* (the Jewish dietary laws), which forbid consumption of pork, shellfish or so much as a cheeseburger with or without the fries. Then there were all the forbidden activities: no drawing or driving on the Sabbath day for it is holy. No coveting of thy neighbour's wife. No showing of one's midriff, bare thighs or shoulders, even in the absence of rolls of flab. The Jewish God seemed to me a 'you-may-not' sort of a God.

A lot like a diet.

After that stormy night when God delivered my parents home safely, I didn't have much reason to call on Him again for some time. I prayed on and off, thanked Him for His grace when things went smoothly as a freshly laid egg and questioned His wisdom and cursed His judgement when they broke like a rotten one. During my early twenties, I delved a bit into Buddhist philosophy and practice looking for ways to still the anxious chicken of my mind.

I was twenty-eight years old when I had my follow-up session with God, which, according to astrologers, is when the planet Saturn completes its first cycle through your birth chart and returns to the spot it occupied when you were born. People who follow the stars claim it as a time of coming of age, marking major personal transformations. Sometime during Saturn's homecoming, I was driving home after three days of meditation and introspection at a Buddhist retreat at Ixopo in Natal, approximately a seven-hour drive from Johannesburg.

To give you some idea of where I was in my life, I'd just said goodbye to my German lover who'd come to South Africa to travel for a year. My dad, whose stepmother's son and husband had died in Hitler's gas chambers (my *zaide* had remarried after

Chaya died), was hoping that I'd just move on and find a nice Jewish boy and settle down. Please accept my assurance that this romance wasn't an act of rebellion against my father, my religion or my ancestry. I really did fall in love with Kurt when we met at a conference with other international lawyers. Why didn't I do the sensible thing and fall in love with an Italian or a Spaniard? I cannot say. Kurt did have very blue eyes. And he was the most ridiculously romantic man I'd ever met. He bought me a rose a day. I know, I know. In any event, my life was more complicated than just a love affair with a German man.

I was at a crucial crossroads in my life and had gone to meditate to try to figure out what to do next. I'd had a great helping of romance and passion in my past (largely thanks to the gorgeous Kurt) and was now ready to move on to having babies. This was an edict direct from my ovaries but the mastermind was, in fact, my heart. I'd been waiting since I was four years old to be a mother and I couldn't hold out any longer. I'd heard horrible things about ovaries drying up over thirty and I wanted mine nice and juicy to make nice, juicy babies. Kurt, however, still had years of study ahead of him, and nappies weren't part of his short-term plans. But Zed, my best friend, was open to negotiation.

I was scheduled to leave the retreat the following morning, having both booked and paid for the Sunday night. However, at three pm on that particular Sunday, for not a single reason I could articulate then or now, I was consumed with an urgent sense that I had to leave right there and then. In the space of an hour I was packed and ready to go. My lovely Buddhist friend Audrey tried to talk me out of going straight away. She had daughters my age, and she didn't think it was prudent for me to drive home so late in the afternoon when I might be feeling tired. Why not wait until the following morning, after

COINCIDENCE #2

a good night's sleep? It made no sense to undertake such a long drive alone so late in the day.

I couldn't explain it. I simply told Audrey I had to leave *now*. 'As long as it doesn't rain, I'll be fine,' I assured her, looking at the clear blue sky before I set off.

The first hour went by without incident. I played my music. I sang aloud. But then the first fat plops of water landed on my windscreen.

Twenty minutes later, it wasn't raining anymore. No, 'raining' is the stuff of umbrellas and puddle-hopping, not the heavens going absolutely ape-shit. In a flash, sweet, loving, aproned Mother Nature turned into a whip-wielding, leathered-up dominatrix. My windscreen wipers trembled and stuttered. The glass fogged up. I couldn't see half a metre ahead of me. I slowed down to a crawl. I murmured, 'Please, please stop the rain. C'mon, this isn't funny ... oh c'mon ...'

I pleaded like this on and off for the duration of that journey, asking God nicely, then imploring Him more forcefully to give it a break. But this time I didn't get what I asked for. The rain poured down unrelentingly. Ten long, eye-straining hours later, well after midnight, I pulled up at my apartment, bleary-eyed with a migraine, where Zed was waiting anxiously. I flopped into his arms, cursing that damn rain.

The next morning, driving out of my building, I heard what sounded like the automobile equivalent of a human limb breaking and my car completely seized up. It wouldn't go forward or backwards. I had to have it towed to Larry the mechanic, who gave me the bad news that the cable to one of the front wheels had completely snapped.

'Lucky you were only leaving your building this morning when it happened. You wouldn't want that to happen on the road at high speed,' Larry told me.

Now at this point, the hairs on my body hadn't quite started to stand on end, but I did say, 'I drove back from Ixopo last night . . . I was on the road for ten hours.'

Larry raised his eyebrows and let out a long whistle.

'And it rained the whole way,' I added, looking for further sympathy.

If this were a movie, this is the part where Larry's mouth might move in slow motion, or a particular eerie kind of music would start to play alerting viewers that this is a pivotal moment in the plot.

Instead, Larry said casually, 'You're lucky. That rain saved your life; it would have kept the wheel cool. By rights that wheel should have heated up and the cable would've snapped at full speed. And that would have been ugly. Someone's looking after you.'

Now all the hairs on my body stood on end.

That rain saved your life.

All the way I'd been praying for the rain to stop.

All the time I thought God hadn't been listening.

That's when I knew for absolute certain that this weird abstract idea of God or guidance or spirit wasn't just a hoax or a trick or a bad ontological plot.

I knew God had been looking after me.

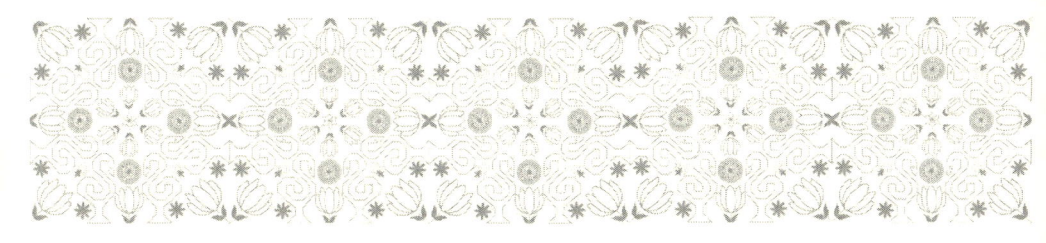

26
God

Man rides, but God holds the reins.
YIDDISH PROVERB

Spiritual experiences, unlike the opportunities a box of popcorn offers, can't be shared. They're as boring as other people's dreams and hopelessly difficult to hang onto. Faith is annoyingly unstable in this way.

Still, I remain quite adamant about God's charismatic involvement in the world, given that fateful drive in the rain. I'm not an advocate of favouritism generally, but when you're the beneficiary, trust me, it's exhilarating. I felt in that moment as if God had shepherded me to safety like a personal bodyguard: 'Excuse me, make way, Joanne Fedler coming through . . .'

I realise this raises the question about where God was for all the innocent victims of airplane crashes, tsunamis and car accidents who don't make it through. I can't answer that. I don't know what God has in mind for other people. My job is to figure out what God has in mind for *me*. Each time I'm spared, I think: I guess I haven't completed what I'm meant to do on this earth, so I better figure out what I'm here for. Almost like I've been given an extension on an important assignment.

There are those, like Richard Dawkins, who have no time for God. I confess that by the time I'd finished reading *The God Delusion* I felt a little dim, like one might do after a particularly rigorous cross-examination where even though you've told the truth, somehow it seems like an incongruous, incompetent fabrication.

I agree with Dawkins that dogmatic religion invokes madness in decent people (not to mention the preposterous obligatory devotional head coverings, veils, wigs and exceedingly large hats). If one couldn't pick and choose one's own wardrobe, life would be a very desolate affair. But it's a little mean-spirited to diss God because of religion. That's like trashing love because of the divorce statistics. Religion and God can sit at opposite ends of the table, like divorced parents of the bride, never once making eye contact as far as I'm concerned.

Dawkins claims those of us who believe in God persist in holding a false belief in the face of strong contradictory evidence. But the question *Does God exist?* isn't the same sort of question as *Does Mount Everest exist?* It's more like *Does Love exist? Does Faith exist?* The answers to these sorts of inquiries, if there are any sensible ones, are surely personal and intuitive, like the colours of jealousy and sorrow.

Joseph Campbell, the mythologist, observed that if we haven't had a mystical experience how can we know what it is? It's like trying to explain the joy of skiing to somebody living in the tropics who has never seen snow. Dawkins may never have had a mystical experience. But, excuse me, what about those of us who have?

GOD

I don't have to see God to believe in God. Like gravity and chemical reactions, there's evidence of God in operation all around me at every moment. I don't know how God works. But I don't see how that matters. I don't, for example, understand how kilojoules, metabolism, parabolas or the theory of relativity work, despite how many times they've been explained to me. However, I wouldn't dispute that they do exist.

I know myself. And I know that it was irrational and out of character for me to insist on leaving that Buddhist retreat at three pm in the afternoon, rather than waiting until the following morning. I mean, I was going to miss *dinner*. All I had was a *feeling* that I had to go *straight away*. I can't explain it any further than that. And in that space, I choose to put God.

It makes no difference to me whether God is an emotion, or a thought or a sense of idealism or indeed the Golem of Prague. I'm just not that fussed about proving that whatever *It* is exists. I am not being facetiously postmodern when I ask 'How do we prove the Truth of anything?', despite the obvious point that we inhabit a post-relativity world. Law school saw to it that I'm familiar with both the rigours and the tricks of evidence, so believe me when I say that what can be proved has nothing to do with what is true. As witnesses for the defence in the case *Does God exist?* I'd call up photosynthesis, Beethoven's Fifth, dawn's first light, breastmilk. Dawkins attributes all these to the law of natural selection. Well, let's not quibble about names. I call that God.

All I know is that when I think about God, there is Something There. It's not a blank. I don't feel stupid or anything. I don't think God is just an Imaginary Friend for Grown-ups. I know God exists.

It's not that I don't want to be an atheist. It's that I simply can't. I cannot, just like I cannot multiply 28,976,434 by

3,875,639 in my head, or run a marathon. My brain and my body can't go there. Being an atheist, in any event, is the soft option. It requires zero effort. All the evidence, as Dawkins states, if we're going to get all forensic on God, points to the fact that there is not, *cannot* be a God. Or if there is a God, he's a psychopath having a laugh (Christopher Reeve is a case in point).

I don't believe God punishes sin (apologies to the Christians). However, I've observed karma's magnificent cyclical dance where wrongdoing comes back to bite people on the proverbial arse. Personally, I prefer 'There's no such thing as a free lunch'. You can call the bill that arrives in the post 'punishment' or 'karma', but you still have to pay it.

I don't know if God answers prayers or creates miracles. For my part, since the rainy night as a child, I have always spoken to God easily, but that could just be me. I can strike up a conversation with an irate teller in the post office just as effortlessly as I can with a three year old looking for fairies amongst the buttercups. It's the most natural conversation in the world to me to address the Great Silence. I also believe that if we pray for the 'right' things, like insight, wisdom and strength to deal with the problems and crises of our lives, then our prayers will surely be answered. Praying to win the Lotto or for a Mercedes hatchback is putting a call through to the wrong department. Isn't that Santa Claus's jurisdiction?

The Bengali poet Rabindranath Tagore in his poem 'Fruit-gathering' writes:

Let me not pray to be sheltered from dangers, but to be fearless in facing them;
Let me not beg for the stilling of my pain, but for the heart to conquer it . . .

Grant me that I may not be a coward, feeling your mercy in my success alone;
but let me find the grasp of your hand in my failure.

In possibly my favourite Bible story, Jacob dreams he is wrestling with an angel on a ladder and when he wakes up God promises him a land, descendants and an abundance of blessings (Genesis 28:10–32:3). And then God says, *I am with you*. 'I will look after you in all that you do and I will never abandon you.' God's promise is not that Jacob won't suffer or never be hungry or feel despair. He doesn't promise that Jacob's heart will never be broken. His promise is simply to be with Jacob – in his suffering, his hunger, his despair, through his wandering, his stumbling, his confusion. *I am with you* (*anochi imach*).

This is as much as I'd expect from a relationship with God. I've never been able to take sweet-talking big-mouths who sprout outrageous promises seriously and I'd discourage my children from dating such people. God's simple promise feels true and honest and right – that when the shit hits the fan (as it will, be assured), God will be there at the end of a prayer. It may not seem like much, but there's nothing that offers more comfort when things go wrong than a hand to hold, or a shoulder to cry on. Prayer, like Prozac, is a management tool. It's there to help us handle whatever life throws our way with grace and wisdom. It may even help us to change our circumstances. But when we can't, as Viktor Frankl, the Austrian psychiatrist and Holocaust survivor, so movingly puts it, 'We are challenged to change ourselves.'

Shortly after Shannon was born, I lay with her, a compact bundle of vernix and tufts of dark hair clasped to my nipple. And I couldn't rationally account for how this moment had come about. Her presence – this fully alive, sucking, breathing little human – was blindingly mysterious and, to be honest, a little freaky. I was taken aback at how little I had to do with it all. I watched her suck, sleep, cry, breathe (how I watched her breathe), and with every inhalation my own importance receded as it dawned on me that I had been an accessory to a silent mystery, a perfect interaction between my body and Some Other Intelligence. It, not me, was the creator. I was happy, if I were to look for a source, to let it be God. Or Mother Nature. Or Sacred Geometry. Or Divine Energetics. But it was surely not simply a chemical or natural force. To suggest that is to miss the poetry of our lives.

Viktor Frankl reminds us that we are a spiritual species, searching for meaning that only each of us can individually craft – and what an exciting and revolutionary proposition that is! 'It' isn't 'out there' somewhere, waiting to be discovered like hidden treasure. We don't have to travel to distant shores or climb the highest mountain to find it. Life's meaning isn't out of reach. We don't have to save up for airfares or frequent flyer points. It's within us. It comes from a place I can only borrow a term for – 'the soul'. I have no idea what the soul is but I know what it's not. It's not my nose. It's not my overweight body. It's not my reflection in the mirror. It's not my law degrees, nor any of my awards. It's equally not my neurosis nor my anxieties. It's a very abstract, non-literal bit of me. The blueprint. It's not anything Dawkins can see or prove or file.

Part of the meaning I give to my own life is to put God in charge. When Zed and I got married, my friend Helen offered to be The Wedding Planner. I nearly keeled over in gratitude

GOD

to her for she is magnificently organised and efficient, and just knowing that someone like her was in charge of making sure there would be enough food, that the wine and the cup and the ring would all be present on cue, freed me up to enjoy worrying about whether my fuschia shoes matched with my purple dress and other such matters of gravitas. She made lengthy lists. She thought of things even I hadn't. The only variable she couldn't guarantee was the weather, despite phone calls to the Bureau of Meteorology. But she had a backup plan – we would move the wedding to her house if it rained. God bless Helen.

I like to think God is a Helen writ large. A force operating with a list of all the things that need to be taken care of in the world, and that I am somewhere on that list. I know that I couldn't relax for a single moment and concern myself with tax returns, leaking ceilings and another infestation of lice in Shannon's thick hair if I thought that the Big Picture wasn't being taken care of by Someone Else who doesn't get as freaked out as I do about parking fines and cockroach poo in the bread bin.

Of course, many people live their lives happily without God, just as I choose to live mine without cocaine or football, which some people swear by. Joseph Campbell said that reincarnation makes possible the idea that there are dimensions to our being and a potential for realisation and consciousness that we have not included in our self-concept. He suggested that our lives are much deeper and broader than we conceive them to be and that what we are experiencing only partially hints at what is really within us. But we can choose to live with a consciousness of that depth.

So there it is: I *choose* to believe in God because it brings a depth and breadth to my life. Without God, I could never have taken the two biggest leaps of faith I've ever made: becoming a mother and boarding a plane with two tiny children to fly to a land I had never seen before and to which I didn't really want to go.

If it turns out that God is nothing more than a metaphor to assist us to work out what we each believe in, that's enough for me. Maybe God is just a notional prompt to support us in getting an answer to the question: *What do you think is possible in your life?*

Some of us need a Buick. Others of us a little rain.

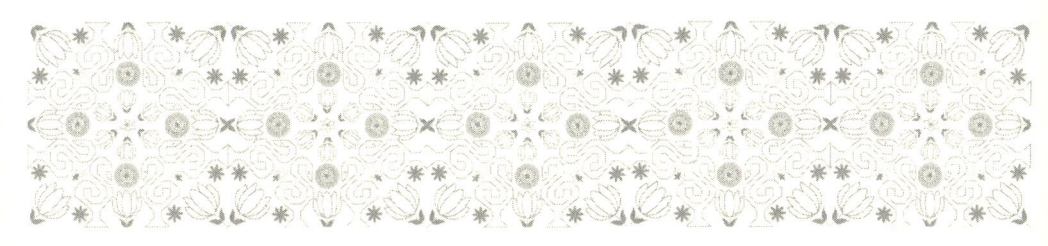

27
Boss

One day of hunger is not starvation.
CONGOLESE PROVERB

'Yuck, I hate tuna,' says Jordan, pinching his nose tight with his fingers and making genuine gagging sounds.

I consider whether there's a real possibility he may vomit all over the dining-room table (he is a vomiter) and then I'll have to clean it up and really, all I want is to eat my eensy-weeny tuna salad without having to handle viscous regurgitation.

'How do you know you hate it? You've never tried it,' I say.

'It smells Dis. Gus. Ting.'

'It's yummy,' Shannon says, tucking into her toasted tuna sandwich.

'It stinks like that smelly cheese Dad likes.'

I won't have a bad word said about smelly cheese. I have a soft spot for a gooey Roquefort or blue-veined stinker. One night in Florence, in the pouring rain under an *impermeable* (plastic raincoat) I was sharing with Kurt, waiting for an outdoor opera to begin, we shared, mouthful by mouthful a baguette, bottle of red wine and chunk of the creamiest, most heavenly, stinkiest gorgonzola between wet kisses. Pongy cheese just makes me think of too much sex in Italy.

I don't divulge this to Jordan and Shannon. They don't 'get' that I had lovers before their dad, and they certainly don't get smelly cheese. Not yet.

'Just as well you don't have to eat the tuna,' I say. 'You can eat your sausage.'

'The smell is making me feel sick,' he whines. 'I have to go outside.'

'Just stay where you are and eat your sausage.'

And that's when he repeats his favourite saying, the one he resorts to when, for example, I issue instructions like 'tidy your room' or 'it's time for bed', which both raises my blood pressure and exacts a mature and intrepid retort from me along the lines of 'I bloody well am'.

This saying is: 'You're not the boss of me.'

Of course, I *am* the boss of him. I am also the housekeeper, disciplinarian, teacher of good manners and fair play, chauffeur, chef and general dogsbody of him. I control his entire life, including his laundry and social engagements, except maybe his thoughts and even those I'm working on to try to turn him into a *mensch* who respects women, thinks war and drugs are stupid and 'gay' is not the worst insult you can fling at someone who wears high pants.

What Jordan's really saying is 'I wish you weren't the boss of me'. It's an assertion of independence, the desire to be free from the tyranny of someone else's rule. I appreciate this longing. I'm working on gaining a little autonomy too.

Recently I've taken to telling my belly: 'You're not the boss of me. You can't tell me what to do.' Food has always had control over me, like a lover who doesn't treat you right and only calls when it suits him. The truth is that hunger and

I have a personality clash. We're never going to be that close. I just don't like what it stands for. Apart from my personal aversion, I also have the tribal issue. Jews are especially not good with hunger. The only time we officially abstain from eating is on Yom Kippur, The Day of Atonement, a full day of fasting from sunset to sunset, the most miserably anticipated day of my year. Nothing is supposed to pass one's lips, including water or fluid of any kind, and for the extremely literal, not even so much as a toothbrush. Of course, on no other day in the year does one think *more* about food or the prudence of a good mouthwash. Deprivation is not the answer to a healthy relationship with food. To make up for this, the rest of the time Jews eat, and we eat a lot.

The Jewish reply to hunger is: Feed it! Have some more! Another chicken drumstick? Have two!

Christianity's response might be: You deserve it! It's punishment for your gluttony.

Buddhism's solution: Be with it. What is 'it'? How is it for you?

The Jewish way clearly hasn't worked for me to date. And I'm so over feeling guilty about food. All that's left for me is to try to 'be with it' and to find out how it is for me to be hungry.

I finish my tuna salad and record it meticulously in my food journal, another entry in this logbook of my consumption, which has become tedious and difficult. How do I quantify yoghurt? In blobs? But there's a discipline to keeping a list. It's one way of becoming mindful and unhooking ourselves from unconscious patterns so we can really see what we're doing. It's impossible to claim 'I didn't know' when you keep a list. A list is a form of personal vigilance, making it harder to lie to yourself or pretend you haven't had that slice of lemon meringue pie when there it is, written for all to see.

A list is a tracking device, even though you might not like the pattern it's forming.

Part Three

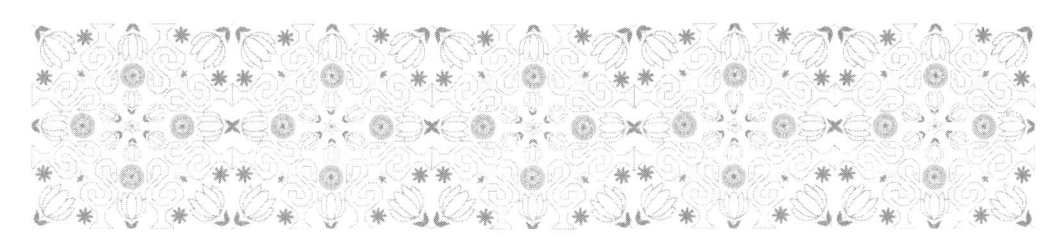

Heartbreak

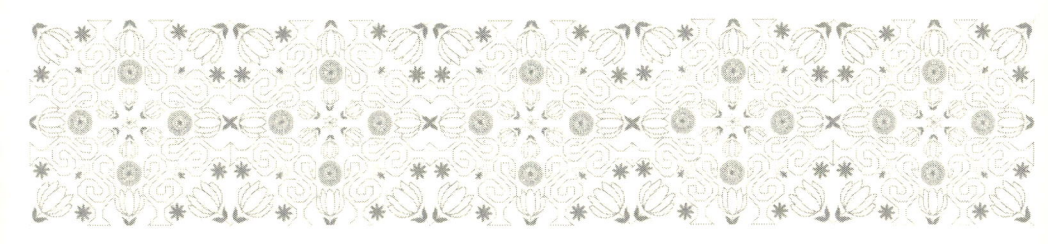

28
The list

The heart is something of a prophet.
YIDDISH PROVERB

Rilke, the Austrian poet, wrote: '*The future enters us long before it happens.*' In Aboriginal mythology, the souls of all things existed in the Dreamtime before the great ancestral spirits turned them into physical beings at the time of creation. Karma, too, is the advent of a future conceived through past deeds. Though I didn't know it, the future had been entering me, dark spirits swarming in my personal Dreamtime, and karma metastasising as I sat at my desk in my cold, poky office offering legal advice to abused women.

By the time I left WAGE to get away from the frontline of face-to-face counselling, my compassion had shrivelled and my patience was in pieces. I was hanging together by spittle threads of anxiety and a neurological lattice of caffeine and headache tablets.

With funding from the Ford Foundation, I set up a legal advocacy centre to end violence against women where I employed six women, including Nthabiseng, Violet's daughter, whose nappies I once changed, as our receptionist. We lobbied (the activist's term for nagged) for more effective laws and trained police officers, prosecutors and magistrates in gender sensitivity, a mission as optimistic perhaps as teaching men how to push in labour. But we were right in there, in the agonising clinch between law and women's lives, doing our best to do some good. During this time, the Minister of Justice appointed me to sit with a group of other activists and lawyers on a law commission committee to draft new domestic violence legislation. Here, at last, was my chance to get it right. I spent a year on this committee working on a kick-arse Domestic Violence Act which was, all modesty aside, a masterpiece. On paper. But without the social and legal networks to implement, support and monitor its pioneering provisions, it was a statutory Tibetan prayer flag. Pity we never thought to hang it out for the wind.

By this stage, I was considered an 'expert', a term which never divulges the desolation that comes with having had your idealism hammered out of you nor the mountain of medical bills on which it rests. I was suffering from severe migraine headaches, unexplained stomach cramps, incessant itching on my arms and scalp and a slipped lower-back disc that kept on slipping. I could discuss the dynamics of abuse or cite the statistics in radio or media interviews. I could talk professionally about how violence was becoming more sadistic – rapes often ended in murder and the age of victims was dropping into infancy because of the widespread belief that sex with a virgin cured HIV. I'd respond to terrible news with professional detachment, but returning home I was unable to relinquish the medical details of some of the cases we'd seen. My mind clutched onto reported fragments and at night I'd toss and turn, the words 'internal bleeding, rupture of bladder and bowel' spiralling like loose balls in my cranium. I could never metabolise the fact of a man raping his four-month-old daughter.

And then the future arrived on my doorstep one day, with a 'Hi, I take it you've been expecting me?' And I should have. If I'd been paying attention, I suppose I should have.

Sandisiwe, one of the women who worked with me, called me at home one afternoon. I took the call with mild irritation – when I left the office I liked to leave my work behind for the day. But this wasn't a work call. I heard the word 'Beauty', in between Sandisiwe's sobs. Adrenalin flooded my veins. I'd come to know Beauty, Sandisiwe's daughter, well. She'd taken to spending the afternoons in our offices studying for her final exams so she could get a university pass and study law, even though I'd teased her she was 'too good' for law. She'd even borrowed one of my dresses for her formal because we were the same size. Sandisiwe's had called to tell me that Beauty had been raped. When I finally returned the phone to its cradle, I stood over Shannon's cot, my hot tears dripping onto her little fists curled in peaceful sleep.

This was a violation of all contracts, an injustice of the blood, a shattering of the vessels of creation. The lines between all things melted. I saw Beauty in the fragile curl of my own baby's body. I addressed God: *Watch over my baby. Watch over her like she is the most precious thing under your care. Do not let harm come to this child.*

The day I found out I was pregnant with Shannon, I started keeping a journal for her. At first it was a list of pregnancy symptoms, then I added my weight gain as she grew inside me and I counted down the weeks till her arrival. Then after she was born, I listed her milestones as she reached them – first smile, first gurgle, first taste of chocolate, first sitting propped with pillows, first unassisted sitting, standing alone, first step – cataloguing all the firsts mothers are obsessed with that add up to a human-becoming-being.

On the day of Sandisiwe's call, I began a new list. Beauty's name was the first on it.

Not long afterwards, an acquaintance of my father's was killed in a hijacking. His name was the second.

My cousin's girlfriend was raped. I added her to my list.

I wasn't with Zed when he got the news that his close friend's mother had been murdered. What you hope for shifts, even in the face of murder. We prayed for a dignified autopsy result. It came back merciless. She had been raped too. I wrote her name down.

My friend Dylan's father was murdered. His name went on my list.

The daughter of one of my father's colleagues was raped. My list grew.

The list became my vigilance, my way of paying attention to what was going on around us.

All I can offer, in the context of this list making, is that it must be a foolishness, a blind, dumb hunger of the ovaries, the same impulse that makes us go back for more chicken soup or another slice of apple tart, that drives the ongoing desire to procreate. The longer my list grew, the more Shannon's presence seemed to give meaning to everything under the sun. If this is sentimentality, and it very well could be, it stems from the human longing for goodness to overcome evil. I wanted another baby. I wanted seconds, to feel the power of creating something pure amidst so much soul pollution.

But like my mother before me who had agonised over my health, and Granny Bee before her, I worried about the world. With every name I added, my growing list was an overwhelming disincentive to have another child, which seemed such an imprudent and selfish indulgence, an unjustifiable genealogical and emotional extravagance. I had no guarantee I could protect the child I had. How selfish to drag a soul by the umbilical cord onto this beaten-up planet and say, 'Make a home here and, by the way, watch out for rapists, murderers and terrorists.'

But Shannon had blasted open the caverns of happiness in my parents' hearts like God's own sweet dynamite. I had never, not even once as a child, witnessed the lavish joy I saw Shannon evoke in my parents. My father said, in a voice fluffy with adoration, 'A grandchild is the greatest love affair of your life.' Two would surely double their bliss. Not to mention all my own unlocked tenderness burbling for a beneficiary.

At the time, Zed and I were living just four streets away from my parents. Shannon spent every morning at my mother's house with Violet, who carried her on her back singing the lullabies she had sung to me and my sisters. Shannon spent every afternoon with my mother watching *Teletubbies* and playing games while I was at work. For the first eighteen months of her life, Shannon was raised in the kitchen of the village of my family. There was so much love to go around, and she grew plump like a little Buddha. This was how it should be. It was a bubble of perfect happiness that was about to burst.

Then, Zed was offered a job in Cape Town. The call of the sea, the lure of that mountain, and the hope of a new start in a new city drew us in like sirens. But it meant ripping Shannon out of the cocoon of love that had nurtured her. Parenthood is relentless in its vexation of the spirit about what is right and what is fair when you're making decisions that affect your children. In a move South Africans call 'semigration', we left Johannesburg for Cape Town, and I saw my mother, the strongest woman I know, cry for the first time ever when we took her only grandchild to a city far away.

In Cape Town, my migraines receded. New life seemed possible beneath Table Mountain, a towering presence that watched over us like God's own level-headed sentry. Under the guardian gaze of Devil's Peak, I grew the courage to go for seconds. Jordan was born into a Cape summer in 1999.

To protect the life we were making afresh in Cape Town, and to clear my mind of the ghastliness I'd seen and heard over the years at WAGE, I stopped reading the newspapers and watching the daily news. I didn't want horror stories to hijack my happiness and blindfold me from the million wonderful things that made up an ordinary day in Cape Town. Like Mandisa, whom I met and employed to be my children's nanny, who was helping me raise my babies. Like the work I was doing with a colleague, Ilze, to re-frame legal teaching full of idealism about how we were going to change the way people practised law in South Africa. Like the Truth and Reconciliation Commission we all hoped would heal the past and herald an era of forgiveness. Like Zed's career which was taking him four times a year to GBDE (Global Business Dialogue on E-commerce) conferences and earning him a shit-hot reputation in his field. Like our middle-class aspirations of some day affording a house. Like our dream of helping Mandisa buy her own home, too. In the meantime, I nagged her to get her learner's licence so we could send her for driving lessons. Oh, I had big plans for all of us.

But my list was growing like a quiet calamity gathering ground.

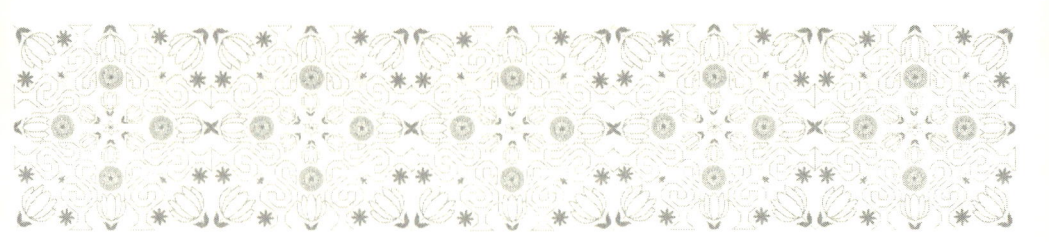

29
10,000 steps

The horizon will not disappear if you run towards it.
BANTU PROVERB

It's nine-fifteen at night and the kids are finally in bed, the dishwasher is loaded and the leftovers wrapped and Tupperwared in the fridge. The surfaces have been wiped down to prevent a cockroach convention in the night. I haven't mopped the floor but it can be left for another day or two before feet start sticking to the tiles. Zed is peeling a banana while asking what I'm doing in the kitchen marching on the spot and whether I intend to be much longer.

'I haven't done my 10,000 steps today,' I say. 'I'm sure this stupid pedometer isn't working. It's been stuck on 5645 for the last ten minutes.' I pull it off the elasticised waist of my pants and give it a good shake. The numbers on the face change to zero.

'Oh crap! I have to start all over again.'

Zed stands and watches me. He finishes his banana and goes for a second, visibly undaunted that he ate Jordan's uneaten cheese sandwiches from his lunch box as a pre-dinner snack, two helpings of my stir-fry, three shortbread biscuits and an apple for dinner not an hour ago.

'Just do another 4355 steps,' he says, showing off how mathematically gifted he is when normal people need calculators for such sums.

'If you don't have anything better to do . . .' I say, wiping a moustache of sweat off my upper lip with the back of my hand, 'why don't you go and amuse yourself by folding some laundry?'

'When are you coming to bed?' he asks, reaching this time for a mandarin. Is there no end to this man's interminable appetite and rapid metabolism?

'When I'm done here.'

'Why don't you come to bed for some exercise?' he asks. 'A decent sexual workover is at least 10,000 steps, probably more. I'll make sure you work up a big sweat.'

'New sheets, I just changed them today.'

He sighs.

'I'm getting weighed tomorrow,' I say, 'I need to work my dinner off.'

'Between your diet and the linen . . .' he grumbles.

'Oh, I'm sorry for the inconvenience,' I huff. 'You might want to let your food digest first. You realise you've just eaten a whole day's worth of kilojoules, right now in your post-dinner snacking? You just stuff whatever you like in your mouth, one thing after the other, no regard for its *schmaltz*, no regard for volume, you just shovel it in . . .'

'I did run ten kilometres this morning,' he says, wounded, between mandarin segments. 'You're welcome to join me . . .' he offers.

'Fuck off,' I suggest helpfully.

'Have we got any chocolate hidden away somewhere?'

'Oh get out of here.'

He opens the grocery cupboard and rummages through a few items before giving up, opting instead for another three shortbread biscuits.

The phone rings shrilly. At this late hour, it can only be South Africa. My father just can't seem to get the time thing straight – he always wants to speak to the kids, but invariably they're in bed.

I hear Zed answer the phone. A moment later he's in the kitchen and hands it to me. 'Your dad.'

'Hey, Dad'.

'What's the matter? You sound out of breath,' he says. 'Are you alright?'

'I'm fine, I'm just doing my 10,000 steps.'

'Your long walk to freedom?' he laughs.

'It's not funny.'

'What happened to your sense of humour? Did you lose it at your last weigh-in?'

'I lost 380 grams last week.'

'Don't lose too much weight, you know how it accentuates your –'

I interject, 'I know, Dad, my nose. Don't worry, I won't lose so much that I'll be all nose.'

'So how are my babies?' he asks.

'They're fine. Jordan got a ribbon at his athletics carnival – he came third in the hundred metres. And Shannon's learning "Bridge Over Troubled Water" on her saxophone. You should hear her, you would be so proud.'

'Oh, let me speak to them.'

'They're asleep, I'm sorry.'

He sighs. 'Oh . . . okay . . . tell them both I love them, okay? Give them a kiss from me.'

10,000 STEPS

I lift my knees. One, then the other. I wonder if I'll ever stop thinking about food. I wonder what would happen if I just made a deal with myself to stop thinking about my next meal. If I did, I may have to think about other things.

Like my friend Ilze's pointing out to me on the phone the other day that my intonation goes up sometimes at the end of a sentence like a real Aussie. Does it?

Like that Shannon was two when she could sing all the words to '*Nkosi Sikelel' iAfrika*', but when I asked her the other day to sing it for me, she said she'd forgotten them.

Like the fact that it's almost a year since my granny died.

Like how I wasn't there when she did and I couldn't be there for the funeral. 'Don't fly back for funerals' had been one of the last things she ever said to me.

I abandon my 10,000 steps to steal into Shannon and Jordan's rooms one at a time, and plant soft kisses on their foreheads.

'This is from your *zaide*,' I whisper.

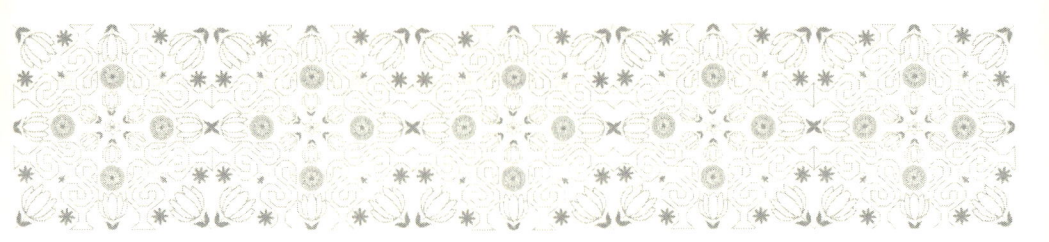

30
Panic

Pray that you will never have to bear all that you are able to endure.
JEWISH PROVERB

While motherhood had centred and defined me, something sinister happened with the birth of my children. I know paradox defines the human experience and romance is always tinged with its shadow, but I didn't expect a visitation from the ugly fairy so soon after Shannon's arrival. The first time I watched her being passed from hand to hand, in her parcel of pink blankets, my chest tightened and no, it wasn't my milk coming in. The shrill sound in my ears and the rapid heart-rate, I soon Googled, were, in fact, symptoms of *panic attacks*. My post-natal euphoria hadn't properly set in before fear sidled up beside it. Jordan's birth had doubled my happiness, but it had also doubled my anxiety to more than the mere sum of my two anxieties (see why maths has always confused me?). I understood how, for many women, motherhood ends up being a case of having bitten off more than you can chew.

PANIC

As long as my children were in my sight, I could pass for normal. But as soon as I was away from them for any length of time, I turned a teensy bit psycho.

Zed and I could be out somewhere having a marvellous evening, doing something ordinary and fun like shopping or eating or watching a movie, and suddenly the normality of it all would strip away unpredictably. A rogue terror reared up inside me, clawing wildly, and I'd imagine something terrible had happened to our children. And then, no matter if our mains hadn't arrived or James Bond had only just been given his mission, I'd beg Zed to take me home.

On these occasions Zed would throw his half-eaten box of popcorn in a bin, or whisper his apologies to our bewildered hosts, and take my hand with the bearing of one assisting a mentally challenged person to cross a road. I could tell he thought I was going crazy, but kindness made him keep it to himself.

One afternoon in Cape Town when I was alone with the kids, I heard 'funny sounds' in our ceiling and grabbed both children and ran into the street screaming, 'Help, there's someone in the roof.' I'd recently overheard that intruders were now breaking into homes this way if they couldn't get in through a window or door. We stood out on the street for a while, with me unable to explain what we were doing to my one and three year old. 'I wanna watch Barney,' Shannon whined while Jordan just cried for his bottle. I wouldn't go back inside until our nanny, Mandisa, returned at five pm and she came into the house with me. After we'd checked for intruders she ran the kids' bath while I made us a cup of tea. She laughed at me until I started laughing at myself.

I'm sure there's medication for this sort of behaviour but I guess no-one wanted to point out that my sanity had gone walkabout.

As incidents like this clocked up, I vaguely registered that hysteria and neurosis were taking charge, like those pigs did in Orwell's *Animal Farm*. I've read enough literature to know that no kid needs a mad mother, if one has a choice in the matter, though of course it makes for interesting autobiography many years down the line. It erodes children's social skills and limits both opportunities for play dates and becoming 'well adjusted', that acme of good parenting. Even if one has superlative communication skills, it's absurdly difficult to explain your madness to your children, so I guess you just end up passing it on to them, like a recipe for chicken soup. Paranoia is both exhausting and demoralising for all concerned, neither is it good for one's health or one's love-life. The eczema I was growing on my scalp was becoming its own ecology and the array of remedies for my unexplained stomach cramps was pharmaceutically impressive. In this condition, you like yourself very little. I sometimes scratched my arms until I bled.

The first time I took Shannon to the movies, she was just two. But as we entered the padded tunnel leading up to the theatre, laden down with popcorn and slushies, she faltered. 'It's dark ...' she said, grabbing my hand.

I assured her there was 'nothing to be scared of' and explained that though it was dark, it was a 'good dark' so we could see better. She loved Stuart Little on the 'Big Scream', as she called it. For years afterwards, she referred to the movies as 'the place where there was nothing to be scared of'.

When she began to name her other fears – monsters in dreams, witches in *Snow White*, wolves and scary forests – I'd

PANIC

paint huge pink word circles around them: 'only a story', 'no such thing', 'just in your imagination'.

I tried to hide my own apprehension with exaggerated efforts to create a perfect world. Along her walls fairies always danced, and in the garden ceramic angels congregated around birdbaths of semi-precious stones. The first and second little pigs in our version, never got gobbled up by the big bad wolf, but escaped to live happily ever after with the smart third little pig, for idiocy seemed a terrible reason to die a horrible death.

But the wheels of my magic explanations that made bad things disappear sometimes got stuck in the muck of my own terror. I couldn't always pull it off, especially with violence and death hovering in the margins of our daily lives. Even so, I could never bring myself to say to Shannon, 'There are some things that are scary and horrible. They give me nightmares too.' I never wanted her to see me scared, afraid it would rob her of her own courage.

So I lied with impunity by day and I think I got away with it most of the time.

But at night, I'd pray, 'Keep my babies from fast cars, drugs, diseases and disfigurement, brain damage and loss of limbs. Give them bulletproof skins and unrape-able orifices, hold them together just as I made them, sweep the world free from all that would hurt them.' I wanted, more than anything, to believe that the world was a place where 'there's nothing to be scared of', and to beckon the simple goodness of those words into the sanctuary of my children's destinies.

Nonetheless, I decided to take action against my fears and enrolled in a self-defence course. There I learned how to puncture someone's Adam's apple with a ballpoint pen and smash their nose with my elbow should such an unfriendly gesture be necessary. Zed slept with a cricket bat next to the bed in case of intruders. Our house was decked out with burglar bars on every window. Every door was doubly secured with a security gate. The bunch of keys I carried around with me could have sculpted my biceps had I curled them repetitively in three sets of twenty. We had alarms installed. I walked through our house with a panic button which, should I press it, would summon an entire squad of security guards armed with guns and batons. It was, you'll appreciate, not a very relaxing existence.

But, say what you like, we were prepared.

Here are some other rules I came to live by:

1. Never wear flashy or expensive jewellery in public. People have their fingers chopped off by attackers if rings don't come off easily.
2. To prevent hijacking, never drive with your doors unlocked.
3. To thwart a smash and grab at a traffic light, never drive with your handbag on the seat next to you. Keep handbags under the driver's seat.
4. Never stop at a red traffic light at night; treat it as a yield sign and, if there is no traffic, pass through it.
5. As a woman, only drive after dark if you have an urgent appointment to be somewhere, like at your own wedding or the birth of your child.
6. Don't stop at night if you see an 'accident' or someone in distress. It is impossible to tell if this is genuine or simply a lure to get people out of their cars. Drive past instead and call an ambulance.

PANIC

7. Don't wear ponytails – they are easily grabbed by attackers.
8. Always carry condoms with you – if you're going to be raped, you at least have the chance of trying to convince your rapist to use a condom, so your chances of contracting an STD or HIV are minimised.
9. Don't open the door to strangers – intruders ring doorbells and claim they are 'delivering' goods.
10. In the event that you are raped, don't put up a struggle. Your chances of survival are better if you 'co-operate'.

With these guidelines as the subtext to daily life, it was difficult to make healthy choices when it came to my thoughts.

There was no denying that fear was definitely the boss of me.

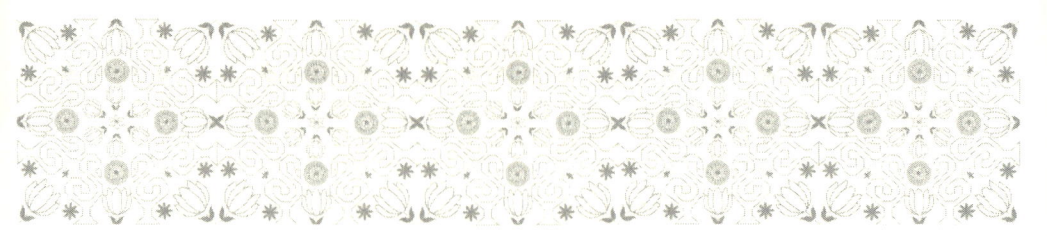

31
Mash

Choosy pigs never get fat.
FRENCH PROVERB

'I cannot eat this,' I announce.

Zed looks at me. 'What, the potato?'

'It's not potato. It's mashed potato,' I explain.

'Yes, I see.'

But of course he does not see. I know this because he helps himself to the huge dollop of mashed potato that has come accompanied with my steak to add to the enormous mound on his own plate.

We're sitting at our favourite restaurant, Five-O's, where you can get just about any meal for five dollars. I had spent at least ten careful minutes surveying the menu trying to decide if there was anything I could order that would not induce an instant conniption in the Food Fascist if she saw it in my weekly ledger, while from all sides the choir of my hungry family sounded, 'Hurry up, Mum, we're staaaaarving'. The choices were chicken schnitzel and chips, beef lasagne and salad, fried fish and chips or steak with mushroom sauce and mash. What you'll understand is that far from appearances, there is in fact, no choice for me on this menu. Everything on it is in *schmaltz*-cahoots to a greater or lesser extent. The Food Fascist has also recently brought to my attention that the average portion size in a restaurant is about three to four times the portion size I'm allowed on my new eating plan. 'The average pasta dish at a restaurant is *eight* half-cup servings. Ten chips is one carbohydrate serving. Count your chips. Don't let a restaurant dictate to you what your portion size should be. And don't *ever* think an eat-all-you-want buffet is a good idea.' Sigh. Of course not.

Eventually, browbeaten by family pressure, I'd ordered the steak, medium rare.

'I take it you want it without the Soddom and Gomorrah?' Zed had asked.

Sodom and Gomorrah is what he calls the sauce, being just a snazzy synonym for extra *schmaltz*.

'What do you think?' I'd grimaced.

The steak had arrived drenched in sauce (despite Zed's assurances he ordered it without) alongside the mashed potato I asked them to spare me. I had tried to request the steamed vegetables instead of mash but apparently the kitchen 'couldn't do it'. Salad only comes with the beef lasagne. I asked if they might just this once pretend my steak was a beef lasagne, but apparently chefs will consider no such sham. *That's an extra five dollars.*

'Don't you want to know why I can't eat this?' I ask Zed.

'Sure,' he says, tucking in.

'How many potatoes do you think have been used to make this mash?'

'Uh, I dunno,' he says, swilling back his beer.

'More than one?' I ask.

'Yeah, maybe.' For someone who can watch a five-day cricket match without a moment's flagging attention, his concentration for such conversations is troublingly limited.

Mash is evil because you never know how many potatoes have gone into your one scoop of mash. If you take a potato and mash it up you will be astonished, amazed and disappointed at how little it yields. To get a decent helping of mash, you need a sack of potatoes.

When you eat mindfully, as I'm doing now, you have to know how much is going in. You can't count something that isn't quantifiable. You can smuggle a lot of potatoes under the guise of mash. There's also a colony of malicious refugees that sneak in with the mash itself – the butter, the cream, the full-cream milk, the cheddar cheese, all harmlessly pummelled into a creamy texture. So it's farewell to the mash, unless I'm happy with a teaspoon of mash, which is, in fact, an entire potato. I'm allowed one small boiled or roast potato. Why? Because it's clear what it is. It is one. One is all I may have. It and it alone.

For this same reason, I'm no longer allowed fresh juices. The Food Fascist almost had a spitting fit when I told her that I 'sometimes' have a fresh celery and carrot juice at a juice bar.

'Do you have ANY idea how many carrots and celery sticks you're consuming in one small cup of juice?'

I'd shaken my head miserably. 'Forty-three?' I suggested.

'About . . .' she'd sniffed. 'I'd much rather you ate a carrot and a celery stick instead of quaffing down a glass which is just choc-a-bloc full of kilojoules and has absolutely zero fibre.'

'Yes, I see,' I'd grovelled, wondering why she insisted on using a word like 'choc-a-bloc' to describe something as un-chocolatey as a carrot and celery juice, which is nasty and bitter and which I don't even like anyway and only ever drank because I thought it was slimming and healthy. Someone once told me eating a celery stick actually makes you *lose* weight because it has so few kilojoules that the kilojoules you use up in eating it makes it a minus-kilojoules food.

But of course, that was incorrect.

The body registers everything we eat, everything we think, everything we say and everything we've lost.

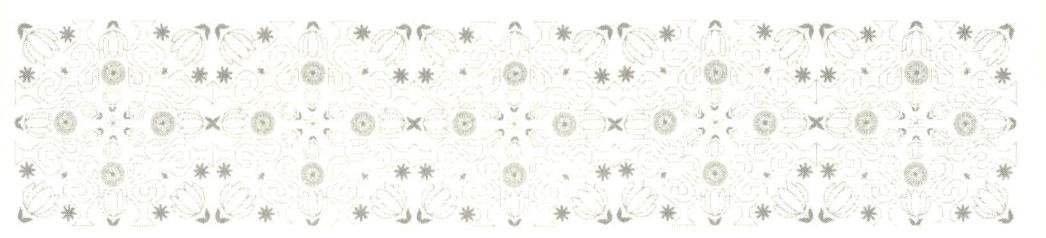

32
The sign

If you really love something, your fate is in its hands.
TUPURI PROVERB

To move on from somewhere when you're unhappy makes logical sense. But to leave somewhere when you're happy is a form of self-sabotage, an existential impudence.

Zed and I were happy in Cape Town. But we were restless. Sometimes we talked about leaving South Africa, weighing up the pros and cons of staying versus going. We tried to isolate and measure the ingredients of happiness, like separating an egg yolk from the white. Personal safety was a good start. But how did it compare with family or balance against kinship? What of history? Loyalty to the country our birth? Soulful friendships? Beloved cats? Woolworths' ready-made meals? The thing the blood does when it hears '*Nkosi Sikelel' iAfrica*'?

If only life was either one or the other, not a perplexing jumble of paradoxes.

This brings me to the question people always asked when I worked with battered women: 'Why do women stay with their abusers?' They'd enquire as if perhaps it hadn't occurred

THE SIGN

to an abused woman to leave, as if the reasons aren't complex. If you've ever owned a small rodent as a household pet, you'll notice they spend a lot of time running around inside a wheel. Once that wheel gets set in motion, it's difficult for it to stop. Abuse is like that wheel, engaging a momentum of tension-building, violence and passionate reconciliation which only sets the cycle off once again.

Abusers, like tempers and bushfires, flare and subside. They're not all consistently aggressive and can be positively charming during the honeymoon phase in the cycle of abuse. Abused women are also hazardously dependant on their abuser emotionally, socially and financially. They often can't see a way out and even when they can they don't believe they'll survive if they go. They stay, too, because of that dogged human trait: hope that things will change.

We stayed in South Africa, moulded to the only contours we trusted, those that held us but that we knew could hurt us. The violence intruded in our lives sporadically, not all the time. We were bound to South Africa in a mesh of emotional, social and financial ties, plaited in with all the clamour and chaos and heartache. We loved the place and its people. Leave? How do you leave your life? Fugitives leave. People who commit suicide leave. How do you abandon your earth, the fixtures of your happiness, the immovables of your identity? How do you disengage from the geology of birthright, where the sky is a signature, and the idiom in which people speak a sacred song of the spirit? How do you start to leave? Leaving is like making the conscious choice to never breathe again. The body doesn't understand the request.

We didn't know how to leave or where to go.

And we prayed that things would change.

I'm now going to go back in time to a moment that changed my father's life and which deeply influenced mine in turn. When my sister Carolyn was a baby, my parents knew intuitively that something wasn't right but doctors couldn't make a definitive diagnosis. Some had intimated brain damage to explain her wild behaviour and failure to speak intelligibly by the age of three. My parents were desperate for answers, and finally scheduled a brain scan for their little girl.

For this, Carolyn needed to drink a full bottle of tranquilising medicine, and the only way to get her to co-operate was to drive her around in the car. So my dad got her settled in the back seat and drove slowly around the block as she sucked on her bottle. All of a sudden, a bird dropped like a stone from the sky, landing feet up, on the bonnet. Keeping the engine running, my dad got out the car, examined the bird which seemed to be dead, wrapped it in a towel and put it on the front passenger seat. When he got home and was walking towards the house, holding Carolyn's hand in his and the bird in the other, the bird shook itself free and flew with great winged gulps into the sky. My father was stirred to his core, believing it was a sign from God that 'everything would be okay'.

Some people don't understand things that aren't facts. My mother's a bit like this, and Zed veers in that direction. People like me and my dad, on the other hand, struggle with the literal, and are much more at home in the abstract and symbolic. After the bird, my father didn't need any more 'proof'. My mother needed the results of the scan. Like my dad, I'm always on the lookout for a sign from God. We're

THE SIGN

not peculiar in this regard. All forms of divination (astrology, tarot cards, the I Ching, or runes) engage with the mystical forces of the universe and have a long history over time. I don't think it matters whether people choose to read tea-leaves, the stars, or throw the bones – it's the impulse to engage the larger realm that helps us interpret the events in our lives. Divination opens a mystical dialogue with the invisible world, connecting us to larger forces in moments of darkness.

Of course, the results of the scan came back showing Carolyn had a hearing problem and there was nothing wrong with her brilliant brain.

After one particular evening of discussion about whether to stay in South Africa or leave, Zed and I reached an impasse – yet again.

'Let's ask for a sign,' I said.

'What kind of a sign?'

'You know, a sign from God.'

'Okay, sure, whatever,' Zed shrugged.

Writing these things down after they happen seems contrived, like a poorly conceived plot. I even doubted myself before I went back to my journal to check.

Exactly the day after we had asked for a sign, we learned that my friend Denis had been murdered. He'd been shot dead at point-blank range on his farm. His eighteen-year-old son had only just narrowly escaped with gunshot wounds.

I never added Denis's name to my list.

I'm not a gambler, and Russian roulette is not my game. I loved South Africa. But it was an abusive relationship. We had to get out. But like the women I'd counselled all those years at WAGE, I didn't know where we could go or how we'd survive if we left.

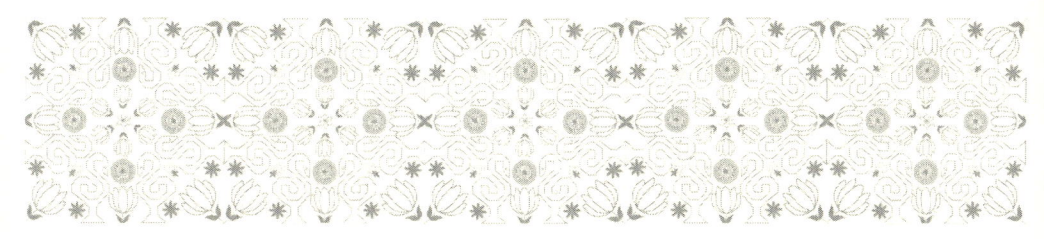

33
Tzimtzum

*God conceals Himself from the mind of man
but reveals Himself to his heart.*
AFRICAN PROVERB

I've heard many lovely birth stories, and I'm very happy for all those women who managed a little squeak and a push and out the baby tumbled. Congratulations, you must be so proud of your vaginas. But for the sake of those of us who didn't score very high in the natural birth eisteddfod, maybe you could play it down a little. For some of us, it was sheer hell we'd prefer to just forget. In fact, if you ask me, it'd be easier to cut labour out of the whole equation and just get on with the job of sleeplessness and bleeding nipples.

During my thirty-six hours of labour with Shannon, my cervix refused to dilate even though this was clearly its job. It just got to three centimetres and stopped in mid-stride like it suddenly remembered something and lost concentration. Even with all the gentle interventions of my midwife, who knew how desperately I wanted a natural childbirth, time passed and still nothing happened. Waters were broken and epidurals administered. More time passed and still nothing happened. So there we were: me on the outside and Shannon on the inside and, despite all the books I'd read, the classes I'd attended and the meditation I'd done, I had no idea how to move the process forward. I thought my body knew how to get the baby out. It didn't seem to. We were stuck. As the hours went by, I started to panic. Somewhere along the way, I forgot I was giving birth to a child and just wanted it all to be over. Thankfully the obstetrician knew what to do. He sliced me open, putting me out of my misery and Shannon into my arms, and if I ever came across another contraction again in my life, believe me, it would be too soon.

After Denis's death, I started experiencing a sensation I can only compare to contractions in labour. I could feel it in the narrowing of my heart and the remorseless spiritual nausea that left me breathless and shaky.

I have to take a big leap into the future, away from that time, to bring some light into what was, undoubtedly, one of the darkest moments of my life. Just like a woman in the throes of labour cannot take in the coos of someone extolling the joys of motherhood, even if I could go back to the person I was and say, 'It makes no sense now, but it will, this pain will pass, and joy will take its place', I probably wouldn't have heard it or believed it.

Ignorance is terrible for many reasons, but largely because information that could bring comfort is concealed. This blindness, which is both terrifying and paralysing, is common in times of spiritual change.

Kabbalistic mysticism explains that God's light is hidden in the world. This stems from the *kabbalistic* idea of creation, in which the first act of divinity was not an outward sign of emanation, as is traditionally understood by the Old Testament's 'Let there be light', but an inward one of divine contraction, known as *tzimtzum* in Hebrew. *Tzimtzum*, according to *The Tanya* (a compilation of *Chasidic* philosophy), means both contraction and concealment, a 'withdrawal and concentration of Divinity into Itself... an act of divine self-limitation as opposed to revelation'.

It makes a kind of sense, don't you think, that if God is infinite (*ein sof*), in order to make space for creation, God had to contract to manifest an emptiness that could be filled. This intense contracted form of original divine light, so the *Kabbalistic* notion goes, filled ten vessels (or *sefirot*), but God's light being so powerful shattered these vessels (*shevirat ha-kelim*), scattering shards of light throughout the universe. Each shard of God's light is now hidden or covered by a shell, and our task as human beings is to crack open the shell to reveal the light. So though God is present everywhere, He is hidden from view in a sort of divine hide-n-seek.

After the shock of Denis's death – he'd been the closest person to me who'd been killed – I felt myself hardening. I was breathless with anxiety about my children. There was no room for the violence to get any closer. In this time of mourning, I wasn't in the mood for a treasure hunt. If God wanted to console me, I wanted it to be easy. I wanted Him to pitch up uninvited on my doorstep with a bunch of my favourite flowers and a vat of chicken soup. Was this any time for God to play hard to get?

The contractions grew closer together and I did forget.

I forgot that even as they feel spiritually obliterating, contractions herald new beginnings.

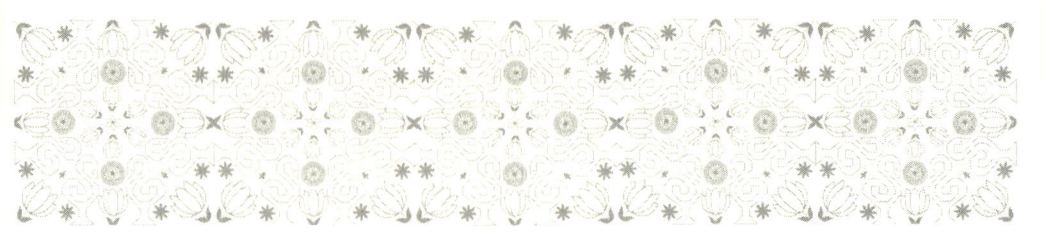

34
Seven

Hunger goes in a straight line, desire turns in circles.
ROMANIAN PROVERB

The Food Fascist assures me that over the past twenty-one days my stomach has contracted. I should probably feel more excited about this than I do. Even if it's true, I still think about food all the time.

I read somewhere that men think about sex every seven seconds. This seems absurd. Think about it – that's around nine times every minute. How might one finish a decent sentence let alone get any work done? Kinsey's *Sexual Behaviour in the Human Male* (1948) revealed that men think about sex a lot though, at least a good couple of times a day. Probably at least as often as I think about food which, even then, is not every seven seconds, but certainly at least every half an hour.

The *preta*s, or 'hungry ghosts' in Buddhist cosmology in the realm between the human and animal worlds, have huge bloated stomachs that can never be filled, and long skinny throats, too thin for food to pass. Symbolically, they represent the insatiable aspects of ourselves, always grasping, always hungry.

SEVEN

The challenge, of course, is to transcend this state. Insatiable hunger — for food, sex or anything at all — is an impossible place of endless discontent.

I've become aware that I often mindlessly wander towards the kitchen or contemplate the nearest place I can pull up for a coffee with a vague 'food' feeling about me. When I get to the fridge, I shuffle jars and containers, looking for something, not sure what. I scan menus and shop counters for a yummy thing. I notice that in the past I've never ordered a coffee on its own. I've always treated it as the beverage sidekick to something else, like an oat biscuit, a slice of banana bread or a muffin.

But now when I order my coffee, an uber-thought intervenes (not unlike those people who push in front of you in a queue): 'Am I hungry?' it says. Then the hungry ghost pipes up. *Who cares? Get out the way. I was here first. Ooh, doesn't the blueberry caramel muffin look good?*

Then that interfering and rather brave new voice replies, 'I care. I asked before and I'll ask again: are you or are you not hungry?'

While the hungry-ghost voice fidgets and tries to push past, the other voice stands firm as my body considers its inquiry. Often, my body isn't sure. It's like Jordan whining at the checkout with a Mars bar in his hand, a muddle of instincts and unbridled emotions. I step in, as the adult taking charge, and drink a glass of water. I check my watch. I'm supposed to wait two hours between meals. If it's only been forty-five minutes since breakfast, I tell myself to wait, even as the hungry ghost whinges that it's not possible that three-quarters of an hour could pass so slowly. This is not the melting of the icecaps we're talking about.

The water shuts up the nagging for a while, but then I find myself thinking about food again.

'Hungry?'

'*Hungry, hungry,*' the hungry ghost shouts.

'How hungry?'

'*Staaaaaarving!*'

'Can you go another half an hour without eating?' I inquire, trying to stretch the ball of my resilience as thin as filo pastry.

'*No, no, I can't,*' the hungry ghost screeches.

I quaff down a cup of miso soup. The tastebuds get a shot of sodium, the brain registers 'stuff's coming in', and this creates a state of temporary calm, clearing a small space I can enlarge by distracting the hunger.

When I find myself thinking about food again, I down another glass of water. By now my belly is a taut balloon. I'm in danger of sprouting leaks if someone bumps into me.

Half an hour and three wees later, I'm thinking about food. Again.

This time, there is an empty gurgling sensation in my belly. A slow sort of growl. Something not dissimilar to approaching nausea.

I pause. Ah, *this* is hunger.

The first time I'm aware of this new experience in my body, I want to celebrate. I'm hungry! I'm hungry!

'*Oh my God. Feed it. Feed it!*' the Jewish mother reflex screeches. And here is where I need to muster a new discipline. There is in fact no urgency. It's just a belly tantrum. Hunger deserves no more attention than Jordan when he's tired or irritable.

'No need to panic,' I tell myself. 'It's okay to be hungry. Hunger is just fat leaving the body.'

SEVEN

When I was a kid, my best friend's grandfather would sit at the dinner table letting out the occasional belch followed by an 'excuse me'. When food was served, his wife, like a withered ventriloquist's dummy, would say: 'Give him a chicken leg. Not too burned. With some potato salad – two spoons. No cabbage salad – it gives him wind. And a slice of bread, no butter. Isn't there margarine for his cholesterol?'

Who knows if the old fella detested chicken legs and longed for bread slathered in butter and a trough of cabbage salad regardless of the digestive consequences? Admittedly, I never once heard him complain. But I also never once heard anyone ask him what he wanted to eat.

It's dawned on me that for most of my life I've treated my body like the old guy. I've never asked: are you hungry? I've certainly never waited for a reply. Instead my brain has spoken on behalf of my stomach. *'It's lunchtime.' 'There's more, I'll have seconds.' 'Ooh, goody, ice-cream.' 'A bit of everything.'*

And like the little old man, I've just quietly shovelled the food in.

All this time, I've been asking like a lawyer. Lawyers don't ask questions unless they already know the answers. It's the basic premise of cross-examination. But this way of asking is a presumption wearing a question mark. Asking like a lawyer is like taking the banana.

There are other ways of asking, like, for example, the Aboriginal way: ask in order to know. To ask in this way, you've got to be able to listen. To listen, you have to shut up. I think that's been my first problem. It's not a path for know-it-alls or people who've 'done the research' or 'been there, done that'.

189

It's a path of serendipity, which could just as easily hook a response from left-field like, 'Bananas are Dis. Gus. Ting'.

I'm going to give it a try.

I make a commitment that from now on, I'm not going to make assumptions. I'll always ask my body, 'Are you hungry?' I will ask in order to know. If I listen, maybe I'll learn something new.

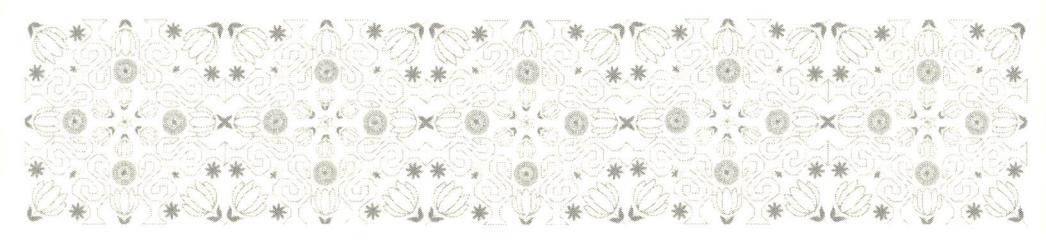

35
Fork

An undecided man is the worst disaster of the village.
NILOTIC PROVERB

Tonight is Zed's birthday and our family custom is that the one who blows the candles out gets to choose where we eat. I don't expect Zed to consider my new regime; a person is free to be as selfish as he wishes on his birthday and endure the karmic consequences at his leisure. He has chosen a very charming pizza joint and has selected the super-sized Carnivore Supremo, with seven types of meat and extra chilli and garlic to celebrate another year of life, though I hardly need to point out that pizza isn't on his biological longevity team. Jordan has chosen his pepperoni pizza and Shannon her pineapple one. Everyone is now waiting for me to order.

Don't get me wrong. It's not that I don't like pizza. I *love* pizza. What sort of depraved psycho doesn't like pizza? However, in the line-up of the World's Worst Offenders in the Fight Against Flab, pizza is a wanton reprobate, it's the Great Gatsby of *schmaltz*-partying, issuing an invitation to every greasy, fat-clogged, sodium-saturated food to perch lasciviously on its crusty, unrefined-flour high-GI base. Hot cheese. Processed fatty meats. Don't be fooled by the veggies. They are just there to tease you sluttily into giving yourself over to obesity.

I am allowed pizza on my new eating plan. One slice.

So please bear with me while I survey the options and decide whether I'd like my kilojoules to come on a triangle of hot cheese with animals, vegetables or seafood.

The waitress's smile is starting to strain. 'You need a little more time, darl?'

'C'mon, Mum,' Jordan prods. 'I'm staaaaarving.'

'I'm thinking . . .'

Zed offers to take Jordan across the road to kick a ball in the park while I make up my mind.

'Oh bugger it,' I say. 'Just bring me a small vegetarian pizza with not so much cheese – can you do it without cheese?'

'Um . . . you want a foccacia – just olive oil and garlic?' the waitress asks.

'No olive oil, just the vegetables.'

'Nah, we don't do that. You could order a focaccia and a salad,' she suggests. 'And put the salad on top.'

'You're a genius,' I blather. 'Yes, thank you, that's what I'll have. With the dressing on the side.'

'Too easy,' she winces, skipping off.

'You better leave her a nice tip,' says Zed.

Give me a break, okay? Choosing a pizza is tough. I'm one of those people who gets in a froth deciding between the Wagyu beef or the duck à l'orange for the same reason that I never wanted to get married. By choosing one, you're saying no to another, and how can one's curiosity ever rest? How do you know if it's the right option? And what if you're missing out?

So please understand that life-changing decisions which herald the tsunamis of destiny are spirit-shreddingly torturous for me. Few things bring us as close to understanding who we really are as a whopper of a decision. To make them, we have to round up all the wise men of our consciousness. We can consult rabbis, priests, imams, crystal balls and astrologers, but, without casting aspersions on the value or livelihood of psychologists, men of the cloth or clairvoyants, we're basically on our own when it comes to picking a path, whether we do it with rational actuarial deduction or by the trusted eeny-meeny-miny-mo method.

As Zed and I stood at the crossroads to this major decision – to stay in South Africa or leave – I was paralysed with fear. What if we made the wrong choice? And how would we know? Could we undo our mistake? If the flapping of a butterfly's wings can create a tornado, what set of catastrophic events would we set in motion by going? I confess that all I wanted was for someone to tell me The Right Thing to do. I didn't want to have to choose.

During this time, I read a lot of self-help books. I came across a quote by Einstein somewhere in which he said there are two ways to live your life: one is as if nothing is a miracle and the other as if everything is a miracle. I cannot tell you how I clung to his words. Einstein was in effect saying, 'Don't get fixated on the *event*. The bird falling out of the sky is not the miracle.' The miracle is treating the bird as a sign from God rather than as road kill. Einstein's insight worked on me, relieving me from the burden of *what* we were choosing and helped me focus on *how* we were choosing.

Zed and I got focused on the 'what' perhaps more than we should have, but through that time we got to know ourselves and each other as moral and ethical beings. At the fork in the road, we ran into the overturned truck of our values, neuroses and anxieties which blocked some roads and opened up new avenues. I had to keep reminding myself to choose the Navman of faith, which would guide us equally on the high road as on the low road. If we chose to leave or stay out of fear, fear would be our companion under Aussie skies as well as under African ones.

I love the *Kabbalistic* idea that we heal the world by making good choices which separate right from wrong. But when in life are two options so clearly either good or evil? The Garden of Eden itself was home to the serpent. Life is nothing if not equally miraculous and shitty. Good and evil are mashed together within every choice. At first glance, this makes things even more difficult — for which one then, shall we choose?

Aha. Does it really matter?

Staying in or leaving South Africa was never a choice between good and evil, right and wrong. But it started a long conversation between fear and faith and ended in an athletic motion, as leaps of faith tend to be.

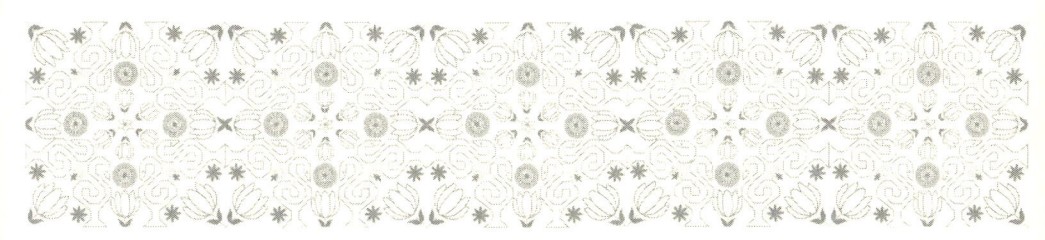

36
Plate

The mouth does not forget what it tasted only one time.
BAHAYA PROVERB, TANZANIA

Zed has a fridge full of beer and a bag full of *biltong* for the rugby between South Africa and Australia this afternoon. He's wearing both his Springbok jumper and a Wallaby beanie. Last year, Zed wore only his Springbok jumper; today he seems slightly embarrassed by the vagueness of his loyalty. After four years in Australia, and with both his children staunch Wallaby fans, he's acquired a dual allegiance which, as far as I can tell, is the best of both worlds, because it doesn't matter who wins, does it?

He's holding a piece of *biltong* under my nose. To get this bag of *biltong*, Zed drove especially to the South African deli in Rose Bay which, Scott who lives in the apartment under Miriam's casually told me, is also called Nose Bay, because of all the Jews who live there. I didn't have the guts to tell him I'm a Yid but c'mon, Scott, *the nose*. And besides, he always brings my wheely bin in for me.

Biltong, like the team you support, is an emotional devotion. It's probably best not to ask questions like 'What am I eating?' because you're likely to gag and retch, like I'd do if I had to eat steak tartar or *balut*, an Asian delicacy consisting of a boiled fertilised chicken egg containing a nearly developed embryo (beak and feathers), eaten shell and all. *Biltong* is a cultural staple of dried, salted raw meat eaten by South Africans from the moment milk teeth appear (my kids teethed on *biltong*), and is a smokeless world apart from beef jerky.

I take the piece Zed's offering and smell it. It's pickled in coriander and meat spice, red and wet in the centre. I salivate a little. My problem is not that I don't like *biltong*. No, my problem is the plate.

One of the Food Fascist's rules is: *Everything on a plate*. Not only must food be on a plate, but one must be seated at a table, not on a sofa. Television should not be involved whatsoever. This is the case even if one is eating nothing more arduous than an apple, which must be cut into pieces and plated up. There's an element of rehab in this.

Eating is an activity unto itself which must not be diluted with entertainment (other than company around a dinner table), nor diminished by the urgency of an appointment or school pick-up. No longer am I allowed to grab something from the fridge on my way out. All these new rules around eating have made it a more demanding experience. But there's no doubt that when you sit and eat something on a plate, you can't pretend not to know, forget or be distracted from the reality that *I am eating*. Once I've eaten, I must then count and record each devoured consumable in my food diary to seal the congruence between what I'm doing and the awareness of what I'm doing.

You don't need to be Steven Hawking to work out that this protocol is both irritating and disruptive of the way things happen spontaneously in real time. These new rules are the culinary equivalent of condoms in coitus, without the rubber aftertaste. But then again, spontaneity is precisely the impulse the Food Fascist is helping me squash when it comes to food. And I've got to admit, it's a powerful counter force to self-deception since human beings try hard to forget what we know, especially when the information isn't comfortable. It's a form of preferred amnesia. I've seen people claim they're happily married while continuing a torrid extra-marital affair. I know others who sing loudest in their place of worship but who do things to small animals or children I couldn't bring myself do to a dead ferret. This ability to bullshit ourselves also explains why theory so reluctantly translates into practice. Knowing is not doing.

Munching a handful of *biltong* during a rugby match somehow doesn't engage the 'I'm-eating-now' consciousness. Which is where the plate comes in. On a plate, eating is eating. Two handfuls of *biltong* are suddenly revealed for what they are: an entire protein allowance of one meal. The plate then, like Pavlov's bell, trains my mind to consciousness. I cannot kid myself that I'm 'just having a little snack', 'whetting my appetite' or 'driving through'. It's this alertness I'm learning to cultivate. The plate is teaching me to be careful.

Vigilance is an acquired skill. And with this in mind, I walk to the kitchen, grab a plate and return to the lounge room, where I put exactly five pieces of *biltong* on my plate, which I will savour while I watch the national anthems.

'Shh,' Zed says to the kids.

As '*Nkosi Sikelel' iAfrika*' starts, a thread inside my heart gets snagged. The lump in my throat isn't the *biltong*. My five pieces are still on the plate.

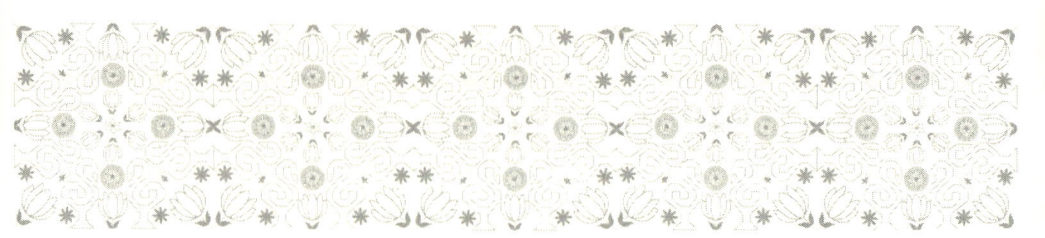

37
A full table

Sweet and sour walk hand in hand.
EFIK PROVERB, NIGERIA

If cities were human, Cape Town would be devastatingly good-looking with that infuriating self-assurance that comes from knowing it's lovable without having to do anything to earn it. I've overheard women say they can't leave a man because he's 'too goddamned sexy', even though he's a rascal and they could do better (I'm quite sure Granny Bee was once such a girl). In just this way it was sheer agony to leave Cape Town because of its beauty. With the sea on one side and the mountain on the other, it was impossible to feel lost, anchored between these muscular landmarks.

During our three full years there, my mother came to visit us every few months. Sometimes we'd drive to Muizenberg Beach to feel the sand between our toes, or to Hout Bay for the fresh snoek and chips while the wind did rude things with our clothes and hair. We had picnics at Stellenbosch wine farms, trailed through the flea markets, and trudged the rugged trails of Newlands forest and the manicured lawns of the

A FULL TABLE

Kirstenbosch Botanical Gardens. One of Zed's sisters lived in Cape Town with her husband and children, so Jewish holidays and family celebrations were always replete with cousins and aunts and uncles.

It's only when you hold your life up to the light, looking for the way happiness moves through it, that you'll see it's kaleidoscopic. It's impossible to distinguish a shard of joy before it shifts like coloured glass, changing every shape and shade with it. What is wonderful in the world is strangely meshed in with all that's terrible too. While I was becoming mired in fear because of the violence in South Africa, I'd never been happier. It makes no sense, I know, but it's just how it was. My life was a paradox wrapped around Table Mountain.

The ingredients of my happiness were many and included the sheer joy of Mandisa. Mandisa was always there with her warm arms when my children cried and when I cried. She never got ruffled when a child had a temperature, attributing it to the spirits of the South Easter. Her presence in our home meant I never felt abandoned to interminable mothering. She shooed me out the house so she could clean and put Jordan to sleep, and I'd slip happily away to silversmithing or writing workshops. She was steady adult company, often the only salvation that stands between mothers and the habit they develop of long conversations with themselves. She showed me the Xhosa way to make *pap* – not thick like porridge, as Violet made it, but almost granular, like couscous, eaten with *amasi*, a sour buttermilk. 'You like?' she'd prod and laugh uproariously when I asked for more.

Mandisa had a thing for shoes. 'Hush Puppy – half price,' she'd tell me, modelling her latest acquisition. She let me know when she thought I looked 'sharp' in an outfit, an appreciation she expressed in a long whistle it's difficult to really describe, but is the singular skill of a tongue that can make those impossible Xhosa clicks.

In Cape Town I had also found Dr Carol Thomas, the gynaecologist I'd always dreamed of (women do dream of gynaecologists and they're women with small hands). She orchestrated Jordan's birth – so it went nothing like the first hell-on-a-drip experience – with my mother, Zed and Thanissara, my Buddhist teacher and close friend, by my side as Jordan squawked his way into the first morning of his life. And she fixed me the tidiest caesarean scar as if she were preparing me for a bikini shoot, either flaunting terrific optimism or an ironic sense of humour.

The violence came in cycles in and out of our daily lives but, during the lulls, life in Cape Town was sweet and abundant, pulsing with the personality of people in sandals who don't brush their hair, grungy earthiness, organic hemp, and men leering out of taxis screeching, 'Hey sexy ...' Everything there made a kind of personal sense, even the chaos.

Living in South Africa was like being in a relationship with Max, an ex of mine who was a mad genius. He might start singing 'Ave Maria' in baritone while waiting for a movie to start, launch into a monologue on Martin Buber with a waitress or enact an obscure neo-Pagan Druid custom while standing in line at the check-out. He was always interesting but, I've got to say, I was never quite relaxed. In South Africa, people spontaneously burst into song and harmonies for no reason but the melody. They dance on street corners, in the aisles of shopping centres, or while strolling through the park. People will never fail to greet you as you walk past. My African–American friend Simone once summed it up when she said, 'African people have fat souls.'

A FULL TABLE

South Africa is a mad hodge-podge of in-your-face opinions and insults, resourcefulness, ingenuity, humanity and humour, in all eleven official languages. Africa's spirit rises from the dust and rains down from the sky, and is crinkled in the dents of old Coke tins others discard as rubbish. I knew, long before I left, as I did when I parted ways with Max, that I'd always miss the excitement, but that staying would eventually bend my mind. You can't get away without adoring such a place, and the more you love it, the more it hurts.

If your heart has ever belonged to someone unstable or self-destructive, you'll know this pain. South Africa is a place of spirit-distorting paradox, a land with a bipolar disorder that swings you from joy to despair in the space of a heartbeat. It twists your arm behind your back and your sanity in a knot. It bullies you until you've forged your opinion on politics, crime, AIDS, the state of the roads, the economy or the politicians. It's not for the wishy-washy or the fence-sitters. It demands you know who you are and what you stand for. It keeps you fit, on your toes and looking over your shoulder. It steals your purse and holds your soul ransom. Very much, I imagine, like being in an abusive relationship with someone both charming and violent. As much as I was, at times, on the edge of sanity living there, I was also stimulated, driven and felt bungy-jumpingly alive. The shades of happiness and fear mottled. I knew that leaving, like chemotherapy, would kill off the best things in my life as well as the worst.

And I had such friends.

Mmatshilo taught me to listen to the voices of the ancestral spirits and to trust that truth has its own power. She showed me how to laugh from my womb, an earthy, rumbling explosion that begins with a long click in the back of the throat, almost as if you are preparing to do a very large spit. Around her neck, beads, shells, bones or other exotic earth-matter always hung as a reminder that she was, after all, a *sangoma* (an African witchdoctor) with a calling to the hills.

'Life is gooooood, Fedlaaaaah,' she'd chant, especially when things were shit.

Lisa is a poet–potter who makes magical lamps combining porcelain and Rumi. Together she and I met monthly to work through Julia Cameron's *The Artist's Way* at Olympia Café in Kalk Bay, dreaming of ways we could truly live like artists. I joined Lisa's ceramics class where I met Craig, a family mediator who shattered every stereotype of men as the emotionally inferior species. But then again, he loves pottery and he is gay.

Craig introduced me to Sherill, a body therapist to help with my back because 'clearly there were emotional issues I wasn't looking at'. I think Sherill fixes pain through laughter, though she did some pretty astonishing things with her hands. I don't know how she works, but she'd touch a muscle and I'd start to cry. In the mystical overlap between the mind and body, she'd tell me, energy blocks get released this way. 'Jo, stay in your skin below the chin. Get out of your head and into your body,' she'd say, as if my head were a building on fire and my body a nice warm bath. I kind of knew what she meant, but not really. When life was unmanageable, she'd say things like, 'Poo is part of the compost of life. We must always include the poo or we miss the lesson.'

Thanissara and her husband, Kittisaro, my Buddhist teachers, soft-spoken outposts of compassionate sanity, directed the traffic of my inner turmoil back to the base camp of my breath. I once confided in Thanissara that I feared I'd lost my compassion amidst all the violence, like a handbag in a crowd. 'Compassion is something we must show ourselves first,' she suggested.

In the afternoons I'd get together with a gaggle of warm-hearted mothers I'd met through playgroups and we'd share coffee and scones and toss our dreams through the sieve of interrupted conversations.

And then there was my friend Ilze.

I met Ilze, an Afrikaans holistic lawyer, when I was doing research to set up the legal advocacy centre a few years earlier – she was scarily smart and seemed so bossy. Over the years, we facilitated workshops and wrote a book together, accruing an intimacy so secluded from ordinary interaction it was as if I'd stumbled into the poetry of friendship. A little went so far, took me so deep, to a place beyond loneliness where I was utterly 'met' by another human being.

Ilze had no habit of reference for things, didn't sloppily repeat other's thoughts or theories, but reframed each situation anew, sifting for karmic patterns. She pointed out that fear doesn't 'happen'. It's something I bring to the party of my own life smuggled in my pockets or under my dress.

'Fear isn't your new lover,' she told me. 'You've been having an affair with fear all your life.'

She also released me from the drudgery of personal explanation. When I was with her, I glimpsed my own spiritual possibilities. I felt truly home.

I imagined our time together was just beginning. But that's a mistake the heart makes, playing with that concept of 'forever' as if it were no more than a doodle on the notepad of life.

Our friendship deserved something closer to forever. But our time had just begun when it was almost up.

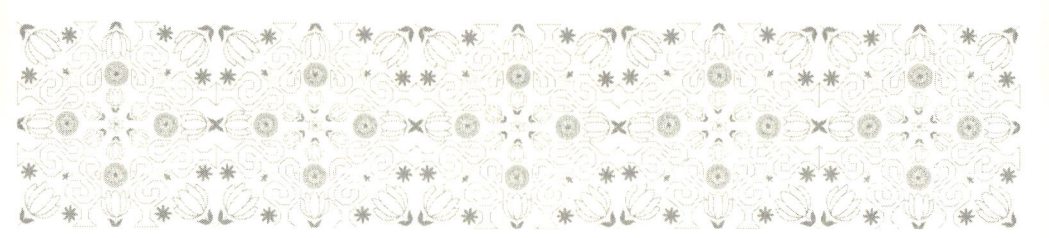

38
Forever

Forever is a long bargain.
GERMAN PROVERB

I'm trying to work on this chapter. But it's hard because it sounds like Jordan has done something life-threatening to Shannon from the screams coming down the corridor.

Is lissom only an adjective, I wonder, or can one use it as a noun, as in lissomness? As I ponder this linguistic conundrum, I hear a thud, and Shannon is calling Jordan a brat, and I can't concentrate anymore.

I sigh and get up. I can ignore this circus for only so long. Unless you give your children your full attention, they will do everything in their power to ruin your afternoon, concentration or peace of mind until you do. Children cannot be fobbed off with fake attention, as in the head nodding, and the idle 'Uhuh, mmm, yes, I see . . .' mumblings parents can make while reading the newspaper, surfing the internet or trying to watch the news.

Even five minutes of real attention suffices. But until such time as you look them in the eye, listen to what they're saying and meet them without evasion in the playground of their hearts, you are a fool to believe there will ever be peace.

'Okay,' I smile brightly as I walk into the lounge room to find the once neatly stacked DVDs strewn across the floor like a pack of cards, 'I'm ready to go down to the beach. Get your scooters.'

Shannon has raced ahead along the footpath on her scooter, while Jordan is pushing himself alongside me. I'm trying to explain the notion of infinity to him since he's just asked me how long it is.

'It's the biggest number you can imagine.'

'Like a million?'

I squint ahead. I can't actually see Shannon, but she can't have gone too far, and she knows to turn around and come back this way once she gets to the end of the beach. She wouldn't have gone into the public toilets by herself . . . would she?

'Much bigger than that, you can't even count up to it,' I say.

'But what if I started counting now and carried on my whole life?'

'Uummmm, even then.' There *was* that child who was raped and murdered in a public toilet in a shopping mall recently. These things even happen in Australia. Where *is* she?

'But what if I'd started counting from when I was born?'

'Even then. It has no ending.'

Jordan doesn't really get it, and I can't say I blame him. I don't really get it myself. Infinity is a koan. The brain can't break it down or work it out. The mind just has to stop trying and surrender to the mysteriousness of it, a lot like we do when we embrace the idea of God.

Okay, Shannon should have come back this way by now. I look ahead anxiously, but I don't see the navy-plaid dress of her school uniform. It's not like I wasn't paying attention, Jordan and I have just been going a little slower. But this is how children disappear, in a moment of lapsed attention. Oh God, am I going to panic?

But there's no need, because suddenly I see her, bright and vivid in the sunlight, scooting back this way with her long hair trailing her. My relief is ridiculous.

I wonder when this anxiety for my children's safety will end. Probably never. My friend Kaaren's daughter is twenty and her son seventeen and she recently confessed that only when her children are both tucked up in bed under her roof does she truly relax. Why do we assume that there are beginnings, middles and endings to all things? Perhaps because life is set up with birth on the one end and death on the other, so we expect all experiences to have the decency to finish at some point. But we're always in the middle – of a relationship, parenthood, housework, a new eating plan or spiritual faith, all of which demand daily renewal, moment-by-moment attention. No sooner are we fit than we have to keep at it or we lose it. The cycle of dirty clothes starts again as soon as it's over. We can't brush our teeth one day and think, 'Well, that's my dental hygiene done'. To be a person requires stamina – the ability to hold the notion of endless cycles in one's contemplation of what it means to be human.

Last week when I went to see her, the Food Fascist made it clear that my new eating plan isn't a quick fix. It's a way of a life, a new lifestyle that must be sustainable. We're talking about forever. The rest of my eating life will be about smaller portions, low-*schmaltz* choices, and no more than two carbohydrates for dinner. I'll never be 'finished'. There's no turning back or homecoming. In this new place of smaller and less, I must find a home.

'Try to enjoy it,' the Food Fascist had said. 'Make each meal a celebration.' (Of what? Misery? Minimalism?)

'Give each mouthful your full attention,' she said, 'like a child that needs you.'

I thought that was quite profound. Just like you can't mother distractedly or half-heartedly and still be effective, you have to eat with your own full attention. Maybe it settles hunger the way it settles a needy child. It reminded me of a woman I once watched with mounting fascination at my first Buddhist Noble Silence retreat who, with Monty Pythonesque caricature, was eating a bowl of rice *one grain at a time.*

Eating is like laundry – it must be done daily. It is like housework – it's never over. It's a daily task requiring daily devotion. But it's also like love. Like prayer. We must return each day, afresh, with the purest of attention to make something beautiful. To feed and be fed.

Later, when I go to kiss him goodnight, I tell Jordan, 'Infinity is forever. Like how long I will love you.'

'Oh, I get it,' he says, threading his warm arms through my hair.

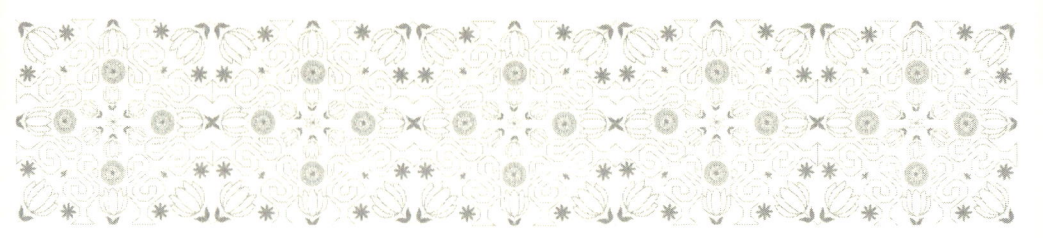

39
Rock

The best kind of closed door is the one you can leave unlocked.
CHINESE PROVERB

'Don't think about it as forever,' Zed said.
We'd agreed in theory to look for jobs in other countries, but we got stuck in two ruts: we couldn't settle on a mutually desirable destination, and the thought of leaving South Africa forever kept clamping the wheels of my brain. Oiling the rust, Zed nipped 'forever' out of the conversation.

'Let's just get out of here for a few years, take a break from the stress. We can always come back,' he continued.

Put like that, I could stumble forward. We could always come back, right?

'Okay, what about America?' I suggested. I'd studied there. I had friends and family there who could put us up. It has Disneyland.

'What about Australia?' Zed countered.

Now I don't mean to exaggerate my own ignorance in these matters, but I think I replied something like, 'Why?'

'They play excellent cricket... and rugby...' Zed said, forgetting for a minute who he was talking to.

'I dunno... I mean, where the fuck *is* Australia?'

Forgive me, but my response was probably warped by an experience I'd had when I was fifteen and on a study program in Israel. What I remember most about my time in Jerusalem, apart from the fabulous bottomless felafel, was an Australian guy, who I'll call Simon. He was slightly podgy with a face like a loose pancake, not that I have anything against pancakes, especially of the low-*schmaltz* variety. But, goddamit, he was so enthusiastic about me and I really needed the attention at the time. I was lonely, on the brink of sexual self-discovery and truly appreciated the way his face lit up when he saw me, how he smothered me with hand-holding and touching of the hair. Looking back at that time, I understand with a shudder why so many women marry the first guy who asks them.

In any event, I let Simon kiss me. It rated pretty low down in my history of passionate encounters, but I did it for what it was worth, and I suppose it went well judging by the size of the erection in his pants. He went back to Australia and continued a torrid correspondence with me punctuated with what became irritatingly recurrent 'I LOVE YOUs'!!!!!!

After only a couple of months of this inane teenage correspondence, he sent a letter which, as it turns out, was the last. After the normal blather about what he'd been up to, he asked if I'd send him a photo. He qualified this by asking if perhaps this could be a naked photo. He then went on to list the reasons he wanted this photograph. Number one: he loved me and was proud of my body and didn't see why we shouldn't celebrate our bodies. Number two: he needed thirty-five photographs of the naked female anatomy for a science project and he had lots of Australian and Israeli girls, but no South African ones. And finally, just in case I didn't feel comfortable about this request, he would be very happy to oblige me with a naked photo of himself, but was courteous enough to warn me that, I quote, 'I have a very large penis'.

None of which, I'm afraid, persuaded me. I replied in a shortish note telling him that girls in South Africa were obviously not as stupid as girls in Australia. That was the last I ever heard from him.

Australia? I couldn't even form a mental picture of it beyond the clichés of desert and marsupials, punctuated with the occasional large reptile. Geographically, bar a few coastal cities, I knew it was mostly desert, an abandoned vacant lot of harsh arid plains. It gave me terrible anticipatory agoraphobia.

But then, in its inaccessible centre stood a sacred monolith of a rock, Uluru. I stared at an image of it Zed pulled up for me on the internet. I know this sounds dramatic, but it was impossible not to feel God's hand there. This ancient, peaceful rock seemed like a sign – you know, in the tradition of birds and rain – an enduring reassuring presence from the beginning of time.

Zed made sure I was apprised of how sunny and beachy Australia was, a land girt by sea, with a fair-sized Jewish population, a stable economy and a thriving democracy. Many of Australia's cities made it onto *The Economist*'s Most Liveable Cities list.

After Zed's Australian PR blitz, my head started going '*Yes, yes, yes*', but my heart was numb.

Three months and two telephone interviews later, Zed was offered a job at a top law firm in Sydney. We had twelve weeks to pack up our lives and get there. Dressed in his best suit, Zed scheduled an appointment with his boss. He returned home that night, tie off and shirt hanging out. Though he's far too cool to actually dance a jig, he was busting to break out. He'd been offered a huge increase if he stayed on in South Africa for two more years. What was two more years? A couple of days, give or take seven hundred. With academic backgrounds behind us, we weren't exactly rolling in cash. And anything we had to take to Australia would be divided by the *tzimtzum* of a merciless exchange rate.

Should we wait, save money, leave with deeper pockets? What would Jesus do? Buddha? My *zaide*? My insomnia worsened. I would have sent a dozen naked photos to anyone who could tell me the right thing to do.

Around this time, I dreamed I was walking along a mountain path, winding my way down towards the valley. I was lugging a heavy backpack, from which things kept dropping out, but I knew I couldn't stop to pick them up. I needed to get down the mountain before dark came and a rising river blocked my crossing. I was anxious about time, but not afraid. When I woke up I said to Zed, with uncharacteristic resolve, 'We're not about money, are we?'

He sighed sadly. 'I thought you'd say that.'

'We don't need money. We need faith.'

'Actually, we need money *and* we need faith,' he corrected me. 'In fact, I'd have a lot more faith if we had a lot more money.'

'We can live on baked beans and cheese melts,' I said.

'Mmm, I love cheese melts,' he drooled.

WHEN HUNGRY, EAT

I entwined myself around the cheeky bastard that morning, reminded of why I love him so much.

We said no to the money. And yes to The Rock.

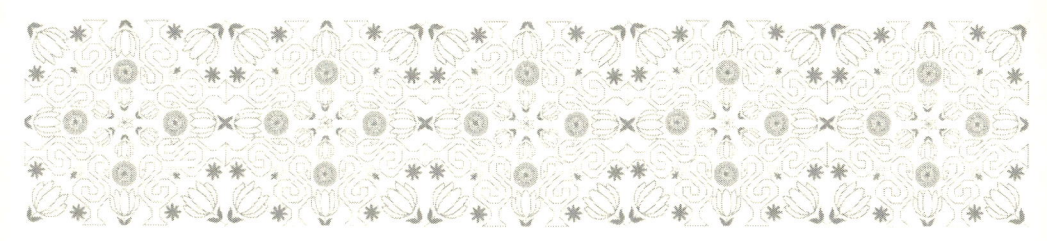

40
Curb

*Before eating, always take a little time to
thank the food.*
ARAPAHO PROVERB

The waitress comes past and asks me (again) if she can get me 'anything else'. I'm sitting at a café in Bronte with the newspaper and a skim-milk cappuccino. I've dropped the kids at school and done an hour's walk, which is only half of 10,000 steps, but I need a little halfway-mark refreshment.

Has she never seen a person drool? This isn't slack labial control or over-Botoxed lip paralysis on my part. I've read the breakfast menu, and I'm salivating over the specials of pesto scrambled eggs on a haloumi stack with aioli, and the smoked salmon and poached eggs with Hollandaise sauce. The old me would have been all over that menu with 'a little bit of this' and 'a side helping of that'. But now I know better. I'd much rather read about than actually wear the haloumi stack.

Looking around me, I see people eating plates of food bigger than their heads, which I now know is not a good thing. I've had my two Weetbix with skim milk already and it's not quite time for my morning snack. I wonder if I'm feeling deprived, and whether I'm hoping someday I'll be able to come back here and order whatever I like on the menu.

I look up at the waitress. The word 'no' perches on the tip of my tongue. God, I find it hard to say *no*. *No* is the word I associate with people like Calista Flockhart or one of those Olsen twins – women who could slide themselves under the crack of a door if, say, they lost their keys. Girls that have no idea how unsexy they look. Those spindly little arms and emaciated faces have been pinched into shape by a million *no*s. No to crispy, no to *schmaltz*, no to seconds. A lifetime of curbed enthusiasm for all things moreish. I just want to see one of them tucking into a hamburger and chips or tub of KFC, I want to see a dribble of barbeque sauce down a skinny chin. Show me one life-affirming *yes*!

I've always treated *no* as the paedophile at the party, the accused in the crime of repression. I've never thought of it kindly or as a word I'd ever want on my team. I sure as hell have never acknowledged its dreams of being spiritually empowering.

But how've I managed to overlook that *no* is the valve that regulates moderation, the core of all spiritual cultures? The human temperament, if left to its own devices, is a slut, prone to an orgy of gluttony, lusts and cravings. For this reason every religion has rules of dietary restriction.

In Judaism, seafood must have scales and fins, animals must have cloven hooves and chew the cud. Only certain parts of the animal may be eaten (no rump, no brains). Meat must be ritually slaughtered by a qualified *shochet* (slaughterer) in a humane fashion with blessings recited. And milk and meat are separated, stemming from the Biblical injunction, 'Thou shalt not seethe a kid in its mother's milk'.

Hindus favour vegetarianism, because of the sanctity of all life. That's *no* to everything with a face on a plate. Muslims celebrate Ramadan, a fast from dawn until sunset over the ninth month of the Islamic calendar, to practise patience, sacrifice and humility.

Dietary laws elevate eating into a sacred act. They are anti-guzzling devices, causing us to pause, much like 'everything on a plate'. When we pause we look again and, in looking again, so spiritual theory goes, we make space for respect and gratitude, which are usually the last to get a seat around the table of a ravenous appetite. Spiritual eating is in fact the art of temperance, reminding us to stay mindful. And *no* is its gatekeeper.

Over the past few weeks of my new eating plan, day by day, hour by hour, I learn to say it, feebly at first, but with ever-greater conviction. No. *No.* NO. Each time I am able to pull *no* out of my hunger-hat, especially in the face of a *schmaltz*y treat, I'm rather astonished to find that far from feeling miserable, I feel pretty powerful. The more I say no, the more I want to say no. Restraint is apparently a muscle you can develop with a bit of exercise.

I remember the Food Fascist's warning: 'You need strength.' I think of my Buddhist friend Taylor, whose mantra is 'Be strong'. And I think of the janitor who watched me and Kurt say a heartbroken goodbye, standing in the early dawn of a Florence morning, neither of us knowing if we would ever see the other again. As Kurt's car drove off into the distance and I sank to my knees in heaving sobs, the old man sweeping the sidewalk raised his fist and said simply to me, '*Coraggio!*' Have courage. Be strong.

I wonder if we're obsessed with the idea that the more you love something, the more of it you must have. Less doesn't need to be a punishment. Saying *no* can also teach us how much we love something.

With this in mind, I turn now to the wisp of a waitress and I let it out, without a tincture of deprivation in my voice, a little burp of temperance. 'No thanks. This coffee is enough.'

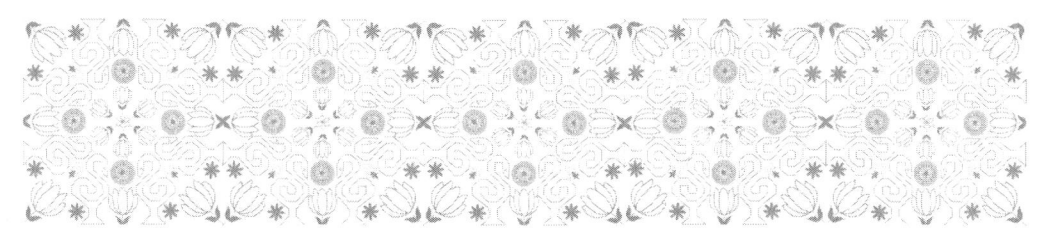

41
Shaken

All things are connected.
We did not weave the web of life.
We are but a strand in it.
Whatever befalls the earth
Befalls the people of the earth.
CHIEF SEATTLE

I was pottering about making the last batch of bolognaise sauce to keep us going for the last four weeks before our departure, wondering vaguely if they have mince meat, bay leaves and Worcestershire sauce in Australia, when my phone rang. It was my neighbour Eunice.

'Joanne, Zed's not in the US, is he?'

'No, he's in Tokyo. Why?'

'Switch your TV on. You won't believe what's just happened...'

I ran to the lounge room with the phone in my hand and fumbled for CNN.

My lack of hysteria surprised me. I'm a drama queen at the best of times. Bee stings. Medical results. Long car journeys (especially in the rain). The red seatbelt sign that comes on unexpectedly during a flight. Phone calls at odd hours.

In this creepy age of live footage via satellites, there on the screen was a flaming tower of smoke, at first mistaken for a horrible accident. An aeroplane had just exploded into the side of a skyscraper that was now burning its smoky wound into the early New York morning.

Then as another plane crashed with deft precision into the side of the second Twin Tower, I wondered, 'Is this real?' And then, 'I should switch that pot off in the kitchen.' And then, 'If this is real, what the hell does it matter if I burn the bolognaise sauce?' Then panic slammed in. Oh. My. God. My friend Adrian, who I'd met at Yale, lived just a few blocks away from the Twin Towers.

With one eye on the TV, I scrambled for my phone book.

I dialled the international code and Adrian's number in Soho. Engaged. I tried again. And again. Engaged.

A slow, sick foreboding lurched in my belly as those towers crumbled into dust.

Days later, we learned that a friend of Zed's, Craig Gibson, never had another morning after 9/11, having arrived on time for his job that day.

After all the anguished terrain we'd crossed to make our decision to leave, 9/11 brought us to a new province of uncertainty.

With just weeks till our departure, insomnia and I took our relationship to a whole new level. I lay awake staring at the ceiling, or maybe through the ceiling, or maybe not even staring at all, holding a hot water bottle to my belly. I thought about my *zaide* and the letter he found the day before he left for Africa. And how he'd folded it and kept it in his pocket, taking it out to read every day on his month-long journey across the water.

I thought of those people – I'm sorry I don't know their names – who jumped from those burning towers. Damned if they did and damned if they didn't. Perhaps when you have no choice you jump anyway.

I wondered why we imagine that it matters at all what we decide. Isn't imagining we're in control of our destinies just a delusion of the human ego? Were Zed and I consciously making a move Down Under, or were we just human petals, falling from a tree God was shaking?

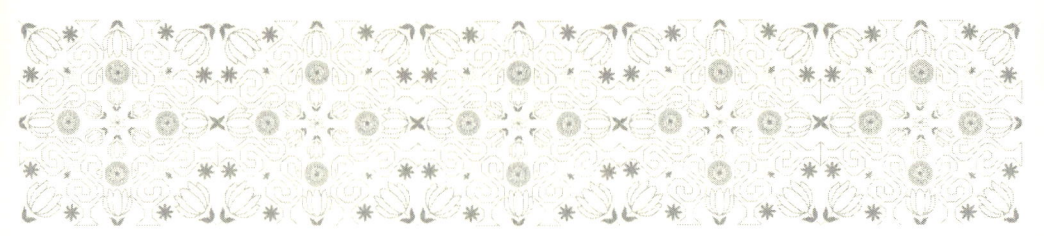

42
Going

To leave is to die a little.
FRENCH PROVERB

I have a special talent. I'm absolutely fabulous at exams and because of this I did really well at school and university. This skill has its downside, though. Once when I was the only student who got a distinction in an English literature exam, I was accused of sleeping with one of the lecturers who, it was rumoured, had slipped me the questions while he was slipping me something else. Thankfully the dean of the arts faculty laughed the matter away. But I have to say, the accusation stung. I really am bloody marvellous at exams.

Despite my skill, if I had to take an exam in 'saying goodbye', I'd flunk. I'm horrible at goodbyes and what's worse is that it shows. I 'wear my heart on my sleeve', as my mother has been at pains to point out to me. 'Hiding my feelings' and 'suffering in silence' are arts I've never mastered. I think it's because I'm a pathetic liar. No, I mean truly incompetent. I'd be a terrible spy. Don't ever ask me to wear a wire. It wouldn't end well.

GOING

It's bad enough that people can tell I'm lying by looking into my eyes, but I can't even lie over the phone. My voice gets funny. I say stupid things like, 'I'm telling the truth', when there's no reason for anyone to suspect otherwise. If I ever have to return something I've lost the invoice for, I get my friend Helen to do it for me, because not only is she an extraordinary wedding planner, she's the most psychopathically genuine liar I've ever met.

One manages one's goodbyes because, like pregnancies, they tend to be sporadically spaced, giving the human spirit a chance to snap back into shape. But when we left South Africa, my goodbyes came all at once. I had to say goodbye to my parents, sisters, niece and granny; Ilze, Mandisa, Sherill, Lisa, Craig, Mmatshilo and Thanissara; Table Mountain, Cape Town; my pilates instructor, writers' group, my gynaecologist, dentist, GP, kineseologist, mothers' group, country, national anthem, work, cats, comfort zone and home. It was a goodbye overload which was all too much to metabolise. Even someone with an extraordinary talent for exams can't do them all at once. Unfortunately there's no 'control–alt–delete' function in the heart, as far as I know.

For both Shannon and Jordan's births, I had caesareans with epidurals. For this, an anaesthetic is injected into your spine which numbs and isolates the pain receptors from the rest of the nerve family while you can magically still feel and move your feet. Then they slice your guts open, a baby is pulled out, you're all stitched up, and all this time you're able to wriggle your toes while chatting about the best place for grilled calamari or a summer vacation.

During Operation Goodbye, my brain did an epidural on my heart. I was numb from my rib cage up. I went through the motions – packing, sorting, getting rid of, selling, making arrangements for, winding up loose ends, executing the million menial tasks that are required when you disassemble a life – but the bits that soften for grief and loss froze. Friends cried during their goodbyes, and my brain explained, 'They are sad.' But sadness had morphed into an alien emotion. My world was being cut to shreds and I felt nothing.

But some nights, Zed woke me.

'You were crying in your sleep,' he'd say.

The logistics of an established life are like tree roots, extending as deeply into the earth as branches reach into the sky and maybe even further, for only the earthworm knows for sure. They are a nervous system, a vascular mesh of intimacies, responsibilities and dependencies, impossible to uproot. The only way to move such a structure is to cut it down. It's a surgical business and sorry, there will be nerve damage. May never be the same again. There are risks with this sort of procedure.

To manage this process, our lives became an inventory. Things to get rid of, things to find new homes for. Things to take with. Things to do. Things to remember. Each 'thing' was the tip of an emotional iceberg. 'Find home for cats' was a blunt headstone for the mountain of grief I had to bury to simply execute this task.

I packed up thirty-four years of my life to *schlep* across the Indian Ocean, every teacup, every paper, every bottle of nail polish I ever owned (and spent the next seven years throwing bits out). 'Will this have significance there?' I wondered about my collection of training materials and South African case law.

I packed it, as I did everything else, *just in case*.

GOING

It's almost a pornography of stationery the amount of paperwork and documentation that's required to prove who you are and what you've done, that you are not a criminal (funny, given Australian history), are HIV-free, can hold a conversation in English and are a decent, upstanding member of society who won't drain the resources of your new homeland through infirmity, illiteracy or larceny. Zed powered his way up the cliff face of certifications, endorsements and authorisations, which at times seemed like a sneaky process of weeding out the weaklings before they even landed on Australian shores.

Adoption always gives me a lump in my throat. No matter how 'unwanted' a pregnancy, I always get stuck on that moment when the baby is taken away from the birth mother. Rationality is a persuasive pimp of sensible choices, but no amount stalls the production of milk in a body that's just given birth. How could adoption be anything but a giving up and a letting go that hurts?

In the weeks before we left, we searched for adoptive parents to safekeep all the treasures we couldn't take with us.

Let me tell you that the problem, 'What will we do with the cats?' is enough to stall the steam train of emigration in its tracks. Should you tell the cats? Do you hope they figure it out? We'd heard of people who put their animals down, but this, like certain sexual practices, was not for me. All it took was for one of our cats to hop on my lap and knead my tummy to cause me to shatter into a broken heap of uncertainties. Eventually, two friends, both devout animal-lovers, took Shadow and Rain in.

It took me days to work up the courage to tell Mandisa. We held hands and cried together. 'Ai, ai, ai,' she crooned, shaking her head. I made promises. We'd find her an even better job. She laughed in disbelief. One couple I interviewed as prospective employers had just returned to South Africa after eight years in the United States, all atwitter with excitement of 'there's no place like home'. None of this was helping. Good people employed Mandisa, but after that I couldn't look her in the eye.

Jordan's wooden cot was given to a friend who was setting up a shelter for battered women. Check.

We dispensed our wooden artefacts and collection of African baskets that Australian quarantine wouldn't allow to whoever would take them. Ilze took a few. It made me stupidly happy to see my things in her house.

Before we left, I sat down to write a letter. 'Dear Shannon and Jordan,' I began. 'Dad and I have made a very difficult decision on your behalf.' I listed all the rational reasons for our move. The violence. The uncertainty. My fear for their safety. We understood we were robbing them of their birthright to grandparents, cousins, an African heritage, countless other legacies of the spirit and the very songlines of their identities. I asked them for forgiveness for twisting their lives away from their source in this tourniquet on African Dreaming. If we were making a mistake, we'd erred out of love. I sealed these letters in envelopes and put them away in treasure boxes for some time in an unknown future.

The packers swarmed in like locusts with cello tape and bubble wrap. I explained to Shannon that all our things would be

GOING

packed into a big box which would go on a ship over the sea and would be there to meet us in Australia. When it came time for our boxes and furniture to be packed into the container, Shannon stood by in silence, watching the whole process with dark, troubled eyes. Finally she sighed discontentedly.

'What's the matter?' I asked her.

'I really don't want to live in that box,' she huffed.

The day I said goodbye to Ilze we stood together in silence.

People assume heartbreak is always romantic with a performance of *Please don't leave me, I can't live without you*, and so on. But the drama of romantic grief has nothing on platonic love's generous sorrow. How much love does it take to bless the departure of those we love instead of cursing our own loss?

Ilze was careful never to burden my grief with her own pain at my leaving.

Finally she said, 'The universe hates a vacuum. Australia is full of wonderful people, go find them.'

'Oh darling, will you really go and live so far away?' my Granny Bee sighed.

'We'll be back,' I told her. 'And don't you dare die while I'm gone.'

'I'll do my best. I'll carry on regardless,' she chuckled.

I didn't look too closely or pay enough attention. I didn't want to know I'd never see her again.

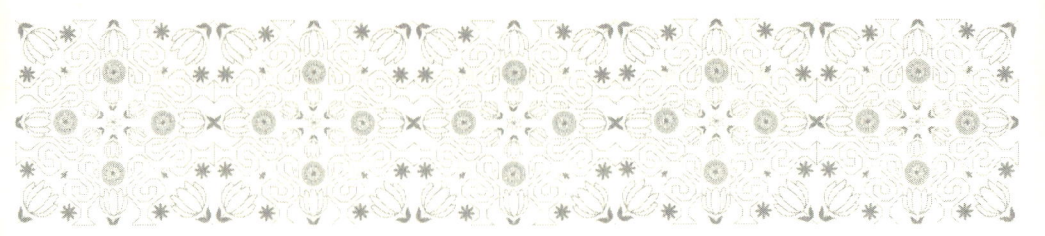

43
Comrades

Tell me your friends and I'll tell you who you are.
ASSYRIAN PROVERB

A pilgrimage from the shores of obesity to the land of 'thinner' is strewn with goodbyes. You have to say farewell to old friends like Vienna sausages, meat pies, lasagne, pizza, ice-cream, chocolate and anything whose first name is 'fried'. Even if they beg you not to go, you should be glad to see the last of them. They're not to be trusted and will pad you in the butt at the first opportunity.

True comrades are rich in antioxidants, fibre, help with the slow release of sugar into the bloodstream, lower cholesterol, reduce the risk of diabetes and are all-round goody-two-shoes in the nutrition department. This may explain why only the vegans and macrobiotic freaks hang out with them. Real friends, would you believe, are oats, low-fat yoghurt, grapefruit, blueberries, salmon, broccoli, green tea, soy and golden flaxseed, some of them sounding more like they'd need to be choked down like malaria medication or fish-oil tablets.

I've personally never had a craving for golden flaxseed. Cravings tend to be for the bad food crowd like chips, green curry, butter chicken, sausages and mash, which, if you fall in with it, will pucker your thighs, lay fatty deposits in your arteries and cause bystanders to look the other way when the wind whips your shirt up on the beach.

But every now and then I think: *Fuck it.*

Even Sandy in *Grease* got to wear tight leather pants and smoke a cigarette. Goodness is tolerable up to a point before we just sicken ourselves with an overload of chastity and righteousness. Jung claimed that 'repressing or denying psychological energy makes it contract into a more intense field', and I say that man understood the simple fact of it: deprivation is the grandfather of failure. To avoid bingeing, splurging and overindulging, I cannot, must not, feel deprived.

If there's anything to be learned from bulimia, it's that the body craves *taste* more than satiation. Lusting after someone, snatching a little flirt or grabbing a quick grope behind the water cooler is often more satisfying than having to take him home, feed him and choose furniture together. Sometimes just a taste is enough.

Weeks into my new eating plan, armed with Jung and the wisdom of lust, I make two independent decisions. Firstly, I'm *not* saying goodbye to any foods. Whenever I want something, I'm going to let myself have it. But only a taste. Not a whole chocolate bar, only a corner. One tablespoon of mash and no more. One bite of a samoosa. Just enough to pleasure my tastebuds.

Secondly, I realise I've been confusing taste and hunger, treating them as if they're one and the same. Though they both speak the language of food, they come from different cultures. Tastebuds are the hedonists of appetite, only interested in a good time. Hunger is appetite's statesman, seeking a solution to emptiness. Hunger is equally satisfied with rice cakes or cream cakes. Tastebuds will try to seduce you into going for the cream cakes. Hunger is happy with the oats. Tastebuds want the Cheesels. Unfortunately Cheesels don't satisfy hunger, so we end up eating more and more and more . . . Tastebuds just want hot sex. Hunger wants commitment.

These are two different needs, and to manage the demands of both, I require a two-pronged strategy. From now on, I will always placate the tastebuds and give them what they want. But — and here's my trick — I will always *feed the hunger first*. This is not favouritism or nepotism. It's a sign of respect. Tastebuds are toddlers and hunger is the adult and adults get served first.

To manage this new approach, I need to know something about GI (glycemic index), the system that identifies the way different carbohydrates give off different kinds of fuel and affect our blood glucose levels. High GI foods release fuel fast, so we get hungry more often. Low GI foods release it slowly and make us feel full for longer. When hungry, go for low. After that, I can have one-night quickies with high GI foods. From now on, I will have an apple (low GI) before I go out to a restaurant. I will eat the broccoli (low GI) before the potato (high GI). Salad before chips. I will only sin after celery.

And I will never arrive hungry at a place I've never been before.

Part Four

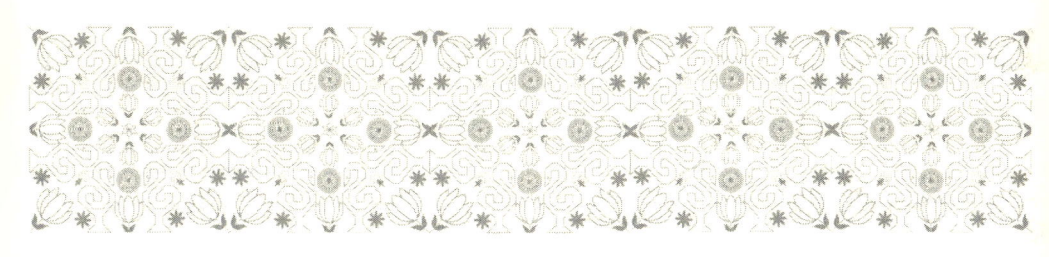

Humility

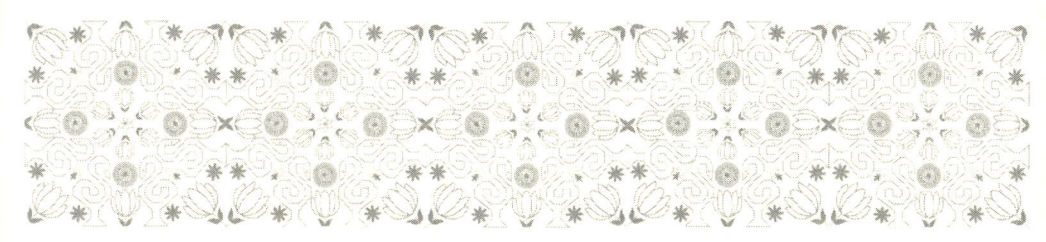

44
Arriving hungry

A foreigner should be well behaved.
YEMINI PROVERB

Down Under. Separately and together, you'd have to agree, these words do not inspire cheeriness. Synonymous with 'depressed', down also doubles up as an instruction to an unmannerly dog, while 'under' is often found in phrases like 'under the weather', 'under the radar' and 'understatement', all rather demoralising as expressions go. I might have been less depressed had our new destination been called 'Up and Over'. But I recognise this is a childish gripe and not one that ought to swing a major decision.

Apart from Simon when I was fifteen, my exposure to things Australian was limited to my Rolf Harris record, gibberished with words like swagman, billabong and coolabah. In my teens the band Men At Work sang of the joys of plundering and chundering, which I presumed were peculiarly Australian hobbies. I thought *Crocodile Dundee* was a great fantasy movie until I saw Steve Irwin voluntarily wrestle a very large reptile on television as if it were nothing more than a beloved, boisterous pet.

WHEN HUNGRY, EAT

A month before we left for Australia, I started reading Bill Bryson's *Down Under*, but the best he could offer in the bits I read was that Australia was 'interesting', an adjective used by friends about men they want to introduce you to when what they really mean is that at your age you can't afford to be too picky. I stopped reading Bryson, worried that it might be making things worse.

It's silly, I know, but I clung ridiculously to the thought that the cartoonist Michael Leunig, a mystical, modern-day prophet Ilze had introduced me to and who draws ducks and a character called Mr Curly, was Australian. You can tell a lot about the soul of a place by its cartoonists.

I stepped off flight QF64 into the inhospitable clinch of a hot Sydney day on 20 October 2001, laden down with two small children and too much luggage and my dear mother at my side. Zed and I had been apart for just over two weeks while he'd gone ahead to find us furnished accommodation, buy a car and settle into his new legal job.

My transition from our life in Cape Town to Sydney was – to be blunt – a mental massacre. I was a ragged mess of emotion before I even got on the plane, held thinly together with the frail assistance of valium and my sturdy mother. The wait at the airport had seemed interminable, with a cranky two-year-old and illegally heavy hand luggage jammed with every item of value I owned, including my jewellery, my grandfather's ludicrously heavy coin collection, cameras and laptop. This kid needed a poo, that one wanted a drink. By the time we boarded the plane, I was a cactus of nerves. The air stewardess prised my pram out of my hands with an undertaking that it would be waiting for me when we disembarked. 'You promise?' I asked with a desperate glint in my eye.

'Absolutely,' she smiled in that psychopathically unaffected way air stewardesses are so adept at.

The sedative I gave Jordan to help him sleep had the opposite effect – I'd been warned there was a small risk – and he screamed and cried and bucked in his seat, but only for the first couple of hours. I got used to the stares of odium from fellow passengers.

When we finally landed in Sydney my pram was nowhere to be found. I wanted my pram. I *needed* my pram. *My pram was promised!* The air stewardess who'd assured me it would be there had vanished, poof-poof, like a puff of two-faced smoke.

As we walked through customs and saw Zed waiting for us I burst, releasing a backlog of tears I'd been holding in for three constipated months. There, in the middle of the arrival terminal, while irritable passengers tried to pass us with their trolleys, I sobbed and snuffled and blew my nose loudly. Zed was here. We were here. We had made it in one piece.

In the car park, Zed proudly presented The Car, a poison-green station wagon. I'd always hated station wagons, with their phoney suggestions of happy families and long car trips, but I'd never been so happy to see one. It was the first thing we 'owned' in Australia. The first claim we could make to something that was 'ours'.

We got horribly lost on the way to our furnished apartment in Randwick. Zed was only barely navigationally literate. No right turn here, nor there, so around and around we drove through dozens of Sydney suburbs, while Zed scanned for remotely familiar landmarks but without a mountain we had no point of reference. I surveyed the passing shops, streets and surrounds with my nose pressed up against the window like an impounded dog, looking for the sunny beaches, the shimmering harbours, the pearly white curves of the Opera House. We passed grubby buildings, several McDonald's, lots of traffic, shops, billboards advertising things I'd never heard of, and people on their way to and from their daily chores. My head ached.

On the kids' beds in our furnished apartment were two stuffed koalas wearing waistcoats that said 'Welcome to Australia'.

'Right, I'm hungry,' I declared. 'What's there to eat here?'

We'd arrived in the middle of Sydney. The middle of what? Was I near the edge, the top, the bottom, the left side or the right side? Which way was the sea, and did this road carry on for a kilometre or a hundred kilometres? Zed drew me a map and showed me how to navigate the two hundred metres to the Randwick shopping centre.

Though I had come from one of the most dangerous cities in the world, in Sydney I was as street-innocent as Chauncey Gardiner in *Being There*, whose entire sense of reality came from watching television. Except in my case, all my knowledge was gleaned from a couple of chapters of Bryson's *Down Under* (who, just for the record, came as a tourist, not a resident), scenes from *Muriel's Wedding* and, even less helpfully, *The Adventures of Priscilla, Queen of the Desert*. Sydney, I should mention, is not for sissies. Big cities shrug off the faint-hearted, the faltering non-native-language-speakers, the on-edge drivers who don't understand why they can't turn right and wince every time someone hoots at them.

A widow should wait a while before getting back into the dating saddle, I recognise this. Likewise, I needed time.

ARRIVING HUNGRY

My first impressions of Australia were made in grief. I spent the first couple of weeks looking for two things: funnel-web spiders and an Aboriginal face, though I never saw either. We drove past the Opera House (*Isn't it magnificent?*) and crossed the Harbour Bridge (*Impressive, huh?*) and the only things I could take in were the traffic and slick hairdos talking into mobile phones. I waited for the *wow*s and the *oh-my-God*s to trip off my tongue – I'm a natural gusher at the best of times. But my gushing had dried up like a post-baby libido. I tried to understand the clouds and make clothing judgements, but the weather often didn't mean what it said. Some days all I wanted was just to dress right.

Officially we were temporary residents on a 457 visa. We didn't qualify for Medicare or free public schooling. We were neither tourists nor citizens, a species half-welcome, half-not.

After three weeks, my mother left and I was abandoned to myself. In those first few weeks I learned that jetlagged children are from hell and nannies are from heaven. I learned that housework is every bit as menial and consuming as feminists have always maintained and that it really is the short straw when it comes to a toss up between the boardroom and the kitchen. I learned that neither my children nor I enjoyed spending all day every day in each other's company. I discovered that TV is a godsend of a babysitter and that people who say children can have too much TV are taking drugs I couldn't get my hands on. Time and again, the kids and I were saved by the sunshine, the parks and *Play School,* an Australian television program for toddlers through which Shannon and Jordan learned about wombats and possums while I developed an unhealthy crush on Jay Laga'aia, one of the presenters. Most of all, I came to realise that Mandisa had been my one and only buffer against the full assault of motherhood. Without her, I was pushed right up against my children, and they against me, in a *tzimtzum* of co-dependency that brings a person most closely up against themselves.

During my tentative forays into public spaces where other mothers stood around with their children, pushing swings and prams, I listened in on colloquial conversations and tried to be friendly without seeming desperate or psychopathic. I found it mentally taxing to join in on discussions about real estate and renovations, topics in which I had zero experience and nothing to add, so perhaps I seemed a bit stupid. I felt a bit stupid and often found occasion to mention that, in fact, I had a law degree, several to be exact, but that made me sound even more stupid. If only someone had thought to ask my opinion on HIV, violence against women, poverty or unemployment. Funnily enough, no-one asked.

Behaviourally, Australia was a world apart from South Africa. In Sydney, it was possible to leave your car not only without a gear lock and steering-wheel lock, but with the doors *themselves* unlocked. It seemed unnerving, perverse even, that you could put your belongings down in a public place and return to find them exactly where you had left them. In South Africa, items bolted down as part of the immovables of your property could be swiped with a little bit of effort and a crowbar. In those first weeks, we accidentally left an expensive football at a local bus stop. Zed went back on the off-chance it was still there and returned with a huge grin. 'This,' he smiled, bouncing that ball at me, '*this* is why we are here.' He was so dumbly happy as if this ball had just vindicated our entire upheaval. But then again, men do tend to value their balls a little too keenly.

In Australia, people picked up their litter and drove at the designated speed limit. I revelled in signs like 'If you dog does a poo, please pick it up', '$200 fine for littering', 'Turn left at any time with care', and 'Turn off engine in event of traffic delays'. Everything was helpful and orderly and serious. Given my own sense of unravelled confusion, I appreciated being told what to do. I needed clear instructions, like those in the early days of a new eating plan. It appeased the teacher's pet in me but upset the artist in me. I did wonder every now and then where the chaos and mess were hidden.

The endless sea of white faces was weird and dislocating after the richness and colour of African streets. I had to force myself not to stare at the garbos, builders and street cleaners who were all white fellas. There seemed to be an economic egalitarianism that swelled my spirit with something verging on hopefulness, that this was fundamentally a good place to bring up your children.

Schlepping kids around by day, I looked for little adventures in conquering new frontiers: Vegemite (Jordan's verdict: Yuck). Fast-food sushi bars (Shannon and I loved them; Jordan's verdict: Yuck). The beautiful parks. The two-dollar shops. The thick weekend *Sydney Morning Herald* with a new Leunig cartoon each week. The luscious beaches. The coffee. The babycinos. We saw kookaburras, flocks of cockatoos and flying foxes, which are in fact icky bats. In grocery stores, we saw kangaroos steaks. We *all* agreed that was Yuck.

For every day the kids and I managed to get through on our own, I rewarded us. Some days it was with a Max Brenner hot chocolate. On others, with a double scoop of New Zealand Natural ice-cream. Some days we'd sit on the beach and eat chips and fried fish, which of course Jordan wouldn't eat due to its Yuck-ness.

'Isn't this wonderful?' I'd sigh with strained cheeriness, to no-one in particular.

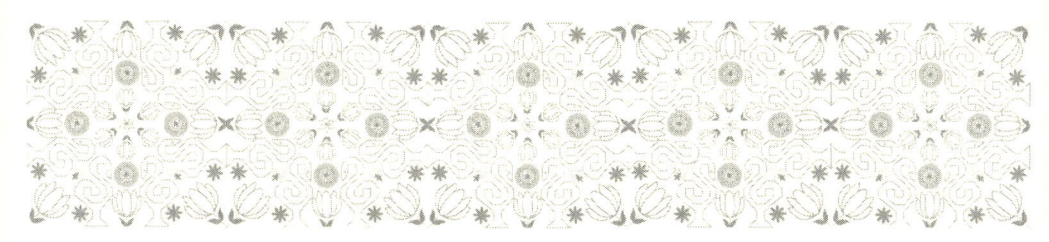

45
Empty

*The beginning of wisdom is to call things
by their right names.*
CHINESE PROVERB

With Jordan in the trolley and Shannon at my side whingeing about the fact that she also wants to be in the trolley and why can't she be, I am, in Positive Parenting speak, deep in the forest of a high-risk activity. Things can get ugly very quickly at 5.30 pm between the rock of two tired, irritable and hungry children and the hard place of grocery aisles of processed sugars.

To ward off any potentially explosive situations, I've taken preventative measures, giving them each a packet of chips to eat while I get our weekly grocery needs into the trolley. I couldn't give a shit if their appetites for dinner are ruined. Rather their appetites than my sanity. But Shannon spots them. Before I can stop her she grabs a packet of Tim Tams and throws it into the trolley.

'Can I have a Tim Tam? Can I have a Tim Tam?' Jordan shrieks.

'Definitely not.'
'I want a Tim Tam!'
'Eat your chips.'
'Can I hold them?'
'I want to hold them!' Shannon yells, fishing them out the trolley. 'I found them, I'm holding them.'
'I want to hold them too!' Jordan screams.

Calmly, I retrieve another packet of Tim Tams off the shelf and give it to him to hold before continuing my grocery shopping with the poise and dignity of one who has cunningly averted a crisis.

God it's a jungle out here.

By the time we're adults with a weight problem on our front and a Food Fascist on our back, we're so deeply immersed in a culture of eating that we have to consciously learn whether a food is a protein, starch, fat or vegetable, just as we only learn 'parts of speech' (noun, verb and adjective) long after we're fluent in our native language. This saturation in both food and language can rob us of our capacity for genuine surprise. It's not often that we taste something for the first time and our tastebuds squeal, 'Holy crap! Get a taste of that!'

But in our first week in Australia, I was smacked with exactly this sensory astonishment over afternoon tea when someone brought out a packet of Tim Tams. Tim Tams, however, ought not to be confused with *tzimtzum*. While *tzimtzum* is a contraction, Tim Tams are very much in the business of expansion, especially around the waist. Tim Tams are an Australian chocolate biscuit that really ought to be nominated for a Nobel Prize for Confectionary.

The way to eat a Tim Tam is with a hot cuppa. Nibble diagonal corners off. Dip the Tim Tam into the tea and suck. Gobble swiftly. Pause too long and the whole melty affair will plop into your hot beverage and you will say 'Fuck'. But if it is fair and right to compare sex and chocolate, this is as good as any rush to any body part that's ever been shown a good time.

The special joy in experiencing something new is referred to by Buddhists as Beginner's Mind, which we can aspire to in all activities – from breathing to walking to eating. To have a Beginner's Mind we have to do a mental spring-clean to toss out preconceptions, judgements, presumptions, histories and experiences we've accumulated which clutter our consciousness and trip us up in spiritual practice. Everything we know (or think we know) becomes a rowdy crowd of know-it-alls, cheering and shrieking instructions, distracting us from what we're doing. If the aim of spiritual discipline is to go further, it makes sense then that there's nothing to be learned from our ideologies, expectations and pre-existing beliefs. Past conditioning keeps us locked in a closet of convention. Therefore, the greatest wisdom resides in uncertainty, echoed in Rilke's words: 'Resolve to be always beginning – to be a beginner.'

My kids used to watch the same *Barney* DVD from start to finish until the sound of that mauve dinosaur singing 'I love you, you love me' drove me to mild electrical appliance brutality. Yet they watched it, laughing at each joke as if they hadn't laughed at it a hundred times before. Children have what adults experience as a mind-numbing capacity to rebuild the same tower of blocks over again with fresh glee each time. What they really have is Beginner's Mind.

Most of our lives are lived out in habit. We repeat patterns without the soul of conscious awareness. When we return to our routines like a beginner, we rediscover the joy, the love and the music that habit has dulled. To start over, we have to have an empty mind. In fact the emptier and hungrier we are the more space there is to be in an experience without prejudging it. We are able to see it, to name it for what it is.

As I learn to be hungry I realise that, largely because of World Vision, I've always associated hunger with unhappiness. I still get very unhappy about starving children, but – here's a new one – my own hunger doesn't make me unhappy. In fact, hunger, like new glasses, makes things very clear. I can finally bring the fine print of my desires into focus and discern whether I want something salty or sweet. Just a taste or something more meaningful.

When I'm hungry, food is sublime in a completely new way.

I stop putting salt on all my food. It's taken me nearly forty years to really taste a tomato for the first time.

Over dinner of pasta tonight, I chew one of my fourteen spirals slowly. I notice that pasta is stodgy. In fact, it's quite gooey and sticky. And I wonder for the first time, 'Do I like pasta?'

If I don't, why do I eat it?

The answer is because I've always eaten it, and because my children like it. One is a habit, the other a sacrifice wrapped in a convenience.

But from the masticating austerity of my slow Beginner's Mind, I have a moment of illumination: it's time to break a habit and cut the umbilical cord on pasta.

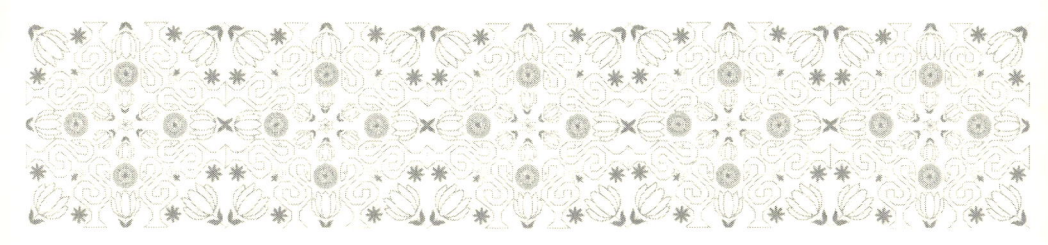

46
Outside

All things grow with time, except grief.
JEWISH PROVERB

I don't recall my parents ever sitting me down to tell me how babies were made. Maybe they did. I do remember a book with pictures in it. In one, a naked man and woman were holding hands, their genitals neatly drawn in detail, lots of hair, the kind of thing you just don't want to see in an illustrated children's book.

I also remember thinking, when the knowledge of how it all happens sunk in, 'They do *what*? Why would they do that? Do they have to? I don't want to . . .' It's impossible to explain to a child that some day sex will be all you'll be able to think about and, for some, every seven seconds.

In my first few weeks in Australia, I was incredulous about all the strange new things around me that Australians took for granted: horseracing, pokie machines, 'No Right Turn' signs at every traffic light, self-service at petrol stations, 'Littering is a Crime' signs, queue etiquette.

As a child and as an immigrant, you're on the outside of experience looking in. Your dispossession from inside knowledge is what defines you. You know the rudiments inasmuch as knowing 'the man puts his penis in the woman's vagina' is an accurate (yet wholly unsatisfactory) description of sex. It *is* that. But it's so much more and it's the gulf between these truths that removes you from participation, always craving a more complete understanding. The only way to get on top of things, so to speak, is with the passage of time, by learning as if you were a beginner.

I came to Australia a beginner, juggling the balls of my own ignorance, a fugitive of competence, and a quintessential *rachmonis*. This is a Yiddish word for 'loser' that comes from the Hebrew word *rachmanut* or 'mercy', because losers are very much in need of mercy. I've always disdained helplessness in others, a trait only hardened during my years at WAGE. But when I arrived in Australia, like Goldilocks, there it was curled under the covers of my personality. And it just wouldn't leave.

I can honestly say (given my sterling record with exams in the past) that I've never had occasion to feel stupid until I arrived Down Under. On Australian soil, I felt like a lumbering imbecile. I lost my way to and from places. I became instructionally illiterate, unable to decode what the traffic signs were allowing and not allowing as if they were written in hieroglyphics. In all my years of driving, I'd never once made an error in stationary judgement to warrant getting slapped with that most pernicious of exploitations by city councils, namely the parking fine. In my first couple of months in Australia, I got *three*. What had I done wrong? The signs had said 'No Stopping', not 'No Parking'.

And everything was so BIG. With over seven hundred suburbs, Sydney tripped my mind. I could visit a different suburb every day for two years. For the first time ever, I felt small. The Sydney Harbour Bridge with its six lanes of traffic was a horizontal Kilimanjaro I couldn't ever imagine conquering. It took me approximately two weeks to establish a square kilometre of competence. Week by week, then sometimes day by day, the circle of my competence widened by metres. (It took me two years to cross the Sydney Harbour Bridge on my own.)

There were practicalities. We had to redo our driver's licences, which meant having to swallow the hubris of all prior decades of driving experience. I passed mine first time (it was an exam, after all). My excitement was slapped down like an alsatian making inappropriate sexual overtures, for there were new rules of the road to be mastered. I was incredibly grateful for small overlaps – Australians also drive on the left-hand side (hurrah!) But *here* the driver and all passengers must wear seatbelts. *Here* the driver must turn and look over the shoulder before driving into the traffic. *Here* pedestrians have right of way. *Here* there are school zones with speed limits that change at different times of the day.

Here you need a permit for that.

Here you need a Tax File Number.

The distance between *here* and *there* became the measure of my personal failings and incompetence.

Zed had to requalify as a lawyer and write a pile of exams. I envied his notes and materials. I was requalifying but without any instruction. I knew how to manage our family affairs and be a mother (I'd been doing it for years without any complaints, right?). Most days I felt as if my skills had been confiscated at Australian quarantine to see if they were full of termites or bugs that could destroy the local ecology. I made mistakes of judgement, wrong turns and deficient assumptions as I bumped my way through each day, dragging my poor kids with me like leaden kite tails.

Sydney was expensive. We hadn't done the maths right. I'd forgotten about 'hidden expenses', and how they are very much, er . . . hidden. Every rand we brought with us was a quarter of an Australian dollar. In those first few weeks I constantly multiplied everything by four to work out what I was really spending. Two dollars was eight rand – I had to stop doing it because I started hyperventilating every time I bought a coffee. It became the metaphor of our emigration: divided and devalued.

Hearing we were 'fresh off the boat', other South Africans invited us for Friday night dinners. We sat around tables of generous strangers, straining for the comfort of familiar Hebrew prayers, accents and chicken soup. Our gratitude was only marred by our *rachmonis* status. There was a terrible loneliness in this, a desperation of spirit in the loss of family our strangeness confirmed. We always arrived with extravagant gifts and laughed too loudly at other people's jokes. Jesus, we were miserable.

We couldn't work out where to send the kids to school or where we should live. We had to make important decisions in a haze of ignorance, as if blindfolded. Friends who'd arrived from South Africa two months before were living in Bronte, so we looked for a rental property there. (Who knew that Bronte is the Hollywood of Sydney?) Our friends had a house. Shouldn't we have a house? They had a garden. Why shouldn't we have a garden? I obviously needed a study. As my *Bobba* Chaya would have said, 'Such greenhorns.' That word – 'need'

– that I bandied about like a birthright was swiftly confiscated, and I have the Australian real estate market to thank.

I had a few truly contemptible encounters with real estate agents, often around the lack of understanding on my part that a fifteen-minute viewing of a property runs exactly on time and only for fifteen minutes. I always arrived late, in disarray, having spent the past hour trying to read a map and drive at the same time with two squawking kids in the back seat. We lost out on a couple of houses because I never arrived on time, nor acted with immediate and decisive effect. Finally, when next a semi in Bronte came up for viewing, I arrived half an hour early; the kids had McDonald's happy meals in their laps, and I zapped my application in before the other prospective tenants had even finished walking through the property.

A day later the following conversation ensued:

'G'day, Joanne. It's Andrew here from BJ Riley Real Estate, how ya going today?'

'Howzit . . . hi, g'day . . . I'm fine and . . . good . . . no worries.'

'Terrific. Well, I have some really great news for you: I'm calling to let you know that your application was successful. The house is yours if you want it.'

'Oh my God! That is the BEST news!'

'Yeah, there were so many people who wanted it – it's a great property, you got in just in time putting in your application so soon.'

'I'm so excited, I just can't believe it. Wow, that's brilliant . . .' (etcetera).

'I should just let you know that the weekly rent we advertised was actually a little lower than what the owner wanted' (intonation rising).

Pause in the gushing. 'Oh . . . what do you mean?'

'Well, we advertised it for $500 a week, but the owner wants $550 a week ...' (intonation rising still further).

'But ... I thought you said we *got* the house?' I said, thinking perhaps 'got' meant something different in Australia, as in 'not got'.

'You've got it ... but the rent is $50 a week more.'

Thus began my initiation into Sydney real estate. We could barely afford $500 a week. But the prospect of repeating the whole house-search, get-your-heart-set-on-something-then-have-it-snatched-away process felt like being told to start labour all over again when you imagined you were home and dry and it was just a matter of tidying up the mess. Zed and I did the maths. We'd have to halve our grocery budget to afford it. So, we'd live on baked beans and toast for a while.

We took the house.

After eight weeks, our container arrived.

With every box I opened, every teacup, every book, every piece of pottery, I rediscovered myself anew. 'This is me ... this is mine ... I bought this at the Hout Bay flea market ... my sister Laura made this for me ... Granny gave me that for my birthday.'

I arranged my history, the accumulation of hundreds of small objects around me as if I was setting a table for a very special dinner party. I decorated my life with my past and, in doing so, I became a little bit more of myself again. A little less of a *rachmonis*.

There are two kinds of people in Sydney: people who own property and the rest of us. Landlords assume the rest of us are filthy, careless, profligate losers who can't even get our acts together to buy our own homes and will therefore trash anyone else's property at the first available opportunity. To curb us renters in our irresponsible ways, there are very strict rental property rules in Sydney. If you happen to be unfortunate enough not to have your finances tied up in a mortgage for the next thirty years, you may not hammer any nails into any walls. Only existing nails may be used to hang pictures.

In our home in Bronte there were six nails in the entire house. Only one in the children's room. We had thirty-four pictures. Shannon battled to pick one for her shared room with Jordan but finally settled on the Flower Fairy Alphabet, though Zed worried about the long-term damage of all those fairies on Jordan's manliness. I gave him the option of hammering another nail in the wall or shutting the hell up. He went for a run instead. I picked five pictures for the house and packed the rest away in cardboard boxes.

I'd promised Shannon a kitten to replace Rain and Shadow once we found a house, hoping a pet would fast track her feeling of 'home'. On the day we navigated our way to the RSPCA in Yagoona, which seemed like another country, there were no kittens ('*Ya shoulda called first, mate*'), only sad cats that no-one wanted. We chose the most depressed-looking of them all, a black-and-white one named Tanaka, catatonic and personality-less having spent the entire eight months of her life in a cage. To have a cat you must have somewhere to keep it, for a cat will not tolerate being toted around in a handbag like some celebrity chihuahua. With Tanaka wandering through the rooms and brushing up against the furniture, we had something resembling a home. There was cat hair everywhere.

After a week of keeping her locked up in the house, we let her out into the garden. She promptly hopped over the fence and disappeared. With Shannon at my side and Jordan on my hip I ran hysterically through the neighbourhood calling, 'Tanaka, Tanaka, come back.' Did she even know her own name?

'My cat's gone, my cat's gone,' Shannon sobbed, and everything she'd lost and left behind was packed into those terrible words. I promised her another cat. A kitten this time. I swore I'd get her one. Tomorrow.

Much later in the day, around dinnertime, Tanaka wandered back in through the laundry door with a look of 'I'm hungry' on her face.

I took it as a sign. She knew where home was. Maybe it would rub off on us.

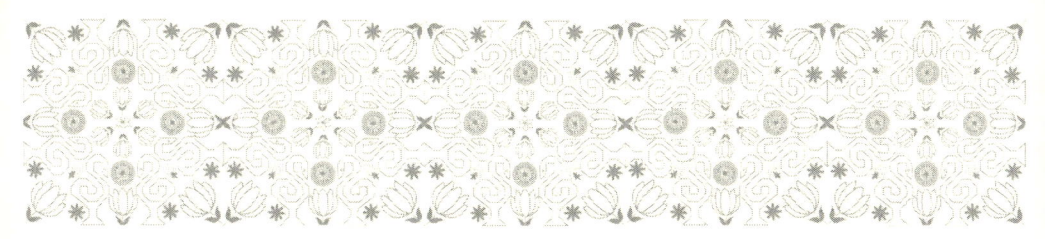

47
Fat cat

A camel does not joke about the hump of another camel.
GUINEAN PROVERB

I am leaning on a metal table. Tanaka is very unhappy with me. She is hiding her face in a corner, as by if doing so she might just convince herself that this humiliating yearly check-up, complete with a weigh-in, thermometer-up-the-bottom and vaccination, is some dreadful kitty nightmare.

But the vet is a large, tolerant man with a mission and, like it or not, despite her yowls of righteous indignation that thermometer disappears up her rectum, yielding a little beep and a normal temperature.

The whole business is over in about ten minutes, but there is bad news. Tanaka is, it appears, overweight.

I pat her sympathetically. With one evil stare she lets me know in no uncertain terms that she wishes to have no more to do with me today and I can just piss off.

The vet tells me I need to buy some scientifically formulated 'reduced-kilojoule' cat food that costs about six times as much as cat food for cats who can wear G-strings in public. I have to give her one-third less to eat. I pat my poor cat again. Oh I know how this is going to hurt.

He tells me that a fat cat is far more likely to get diabetes and that is no fun for all concerned. I have to make sure she loses weight.

As he leaves the room to get me a bag of ridiculously priced feline Lean Cuisine, I notice a poster on the wall next to the bottles of unguents for infected animal wounds: *Does your dog suffer from weeping pustules and itchy red rashes? It could be due to the Wandering Jew.*

My God! Are these types of posters even *allowed*? Isn't there a law against this sort of thing? Various international conventions?

Australia is, overall, a tolerant country, a blend of religions and languages and colours and communities with a thriving Jewish community that embraces all newcomers. When we arrived, I was bowled over by a big basket of goodies that was delivered to our door from the South African Jewish something or other. How did they even know we were here?

But like in all countries, there is underlying racism, homophobia and anti-Semitism and this poster is just a little unsubtle. Just as I'm bundling my butterball of a pet into her basket and stomping out, I discover, by reading the small print that's not really so small, that Wandering Jew is, it appears, a succulent creeping plant native to South America that's 'popular in gardens as a groundcover and establishes easily in moist shady areas. It spreads quickly and out-competes other native vegetation.'

I wonder momentarily if there's anything to be offended by here. Is this a subtle way of saying, via a seemingly innocuous vegetation wall chart, that Jews take over wherever we go?

I feel wounded. I look at Tanaka's yellow eyes. She looks wounded too.

At least Tanaka can get away with anonymity in the religion department. But like me, she's going to be hungry for a while to come.

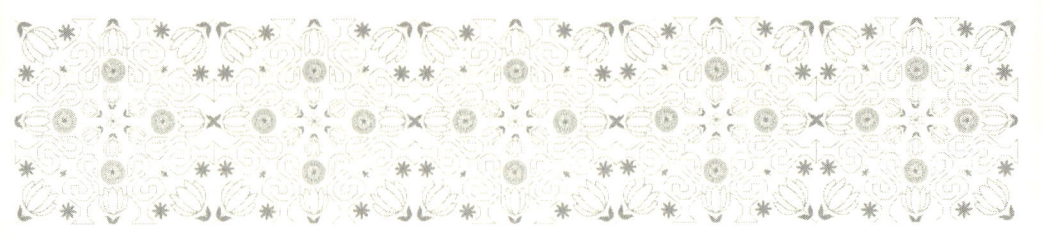

48
Extra virgin

The beginning is the half of every action.
GREEK PROVERB

When you're hungry, a pickle helps – which is why I always keep a jar in the fridge. My granny used to make pickles. This involved her boiling up a brew of vinegar, sugar, bay leaves, peppercorns, salt and coriander seeds, which she'd pour over sliced cucumbers, carrots, cauliflower and red peppers. The veggies then had to 'sit' in the brine in their glass jars to get that pickled flavour. 'You cannot rush a pickle,' my granny would say.

She was right. If you eat a pickle too soon, it's neither fresh nor pickled but instead something uncertain, in between, that you'd really rather spit out than swallow. When it comes to pickling, patience and osmosis do all the work.

'Culture shock' is a scalding jolt, like hot brine poured over veggies. No urgency or impatience can fast forward the slow marinating of acclimatisation. Only when you've been in a place long enough will the culture, history and social norms seep in, like dreams on the outside, to cure you properly.

There is a lesson in love here that I've heard expressed as 'You only know what you've got when it's gone'. We don't experience the myriad social, cultural and political forces that define us – whether to greet strangers, whether it's acceptable to leave the house in flip-flops and a singlet, what newspaper to read, how to ask for directions – as bodies of knowledge to imbibe. We know what to do. We don't acknowledge gravity or oxygen as forces to come to terms with until we're underwater or hurtling through space. We don't have to remind ourselves to breathe or to stand up straight. The human body has involuntary reflexes that kick in.

When I arrived, I often had to remind myself to breathe.

In Australia, the days dripped into me one by one. I discovered a new way of talking. I picked up discards of conversations, like a seagull raiding the picnic site: EFTPOS, Medicare, flat white, super fund, DOCS, Anzac Day, true blue, bogan, AFL, bludger, Tatts. I listened to the things people said and how they said them. I needed time to sit in Australian humour and idiom, social customs, talkback radio and television so I could learn to laugh, joke and banter afresh.

I quickly learned to swap my instinctive 'Ja' for 'Yeah'. I tried with the concentration of a stutterer not to say, 'Howzit?' and 'Good – and you?' and tried out 'G'day, mate' and 'Yeah, I'm awright'. I stalked phrases, waiting for a chance to use them. I desperately wanted an opportunity to say 'no worries'. I listened, but it took a while before I heard an Aussie actually say 'fair dinkum'. I did once hear someone machete English grammar by putting a 'but' at the end of a sentence, as in, 'I don't think so, but'.

Here's what I noticed: Aussies tend to intonate upwards instead of downwards, as if each sentence is arching towards a question. They shorten things: brekkie for breakfast, footie for football, garbo for garbageman, arvo for afternoon, chook for chicken. I worried that this *meant* something, perhaps an ontological fallout of *tzimtzum* or spiritual reduction. Australians really pronounce their Is in words like milk, so when I asked for 'mulk' in my coffee, baristas looked at me oddly, as if I'd asked for turtle brains. My tongue craved the easy thickness of South African phrases. I phoned Ilze just to hear her Afrikaans accent, revelling in the rolling Rs that trilled in my mouth and the gentle switch between English and Afrikaans phrases: 'Howzit, my friend? *Hoe gaan dit? Ja*, we're *lekka . . .*'

Whenever I'd hear another South African accent I'd turn to it like a mother to her baby's cry. I'd want to hug this stranger who spoke like me.

'How long have you been here?' is a dead giveaway that you're raw. How long? It became my silliness. I learned that South Africans who've been here more than two years don't measure that space anymore, just like we stop counting in days, then in months the ages of our children. I envied these veteran immigrants with ten, fifteen years under their belts. I coveted their ease, as a novice doing dog paddle might feel about Ian Thorpe doing laps in the next lane.

I didn't understand that I was metabolising loss.

I am alone, I am lost. I wanted to weep at every ordinary encounter: a waitress serving me a toasted sandwich, someone cutting me off in the traffic. I am alone. I am lost. It was so strong in me, I was sure people could smell it.

'Do you want a sugar with that?' *I am lost. I am alone.* It was the answer to every question.

There was a perfection to this loss. It suffused my existence, radiating through me. My competence in matters I'd once been so confident with disintegrated, a tissue of self-delusion. I got lost in the aisles looking for the tomato sauce. When I found it, there were seven different kinds, none of which I recognised. Which one would Shannon eat? Making small talk. I sounded ridiculous, trying too hard.

For the first few months I didn't understand a thing except *Big Brother*, which seems to be the same everywhere in the world. I watched it greedily every night. It became my obsession.

I said 'I'm sorry' a lot.

I had only expressed it a few times, how much I craved to be 'rooted' in Australia, before someone kindly pointed out to me that in Australia 'root' is a colloquialism for 'fuck'.

I stumbled into an episode of *Kath & Kim*, not sure if it was reality TV or a satire.

I was shocked by some of the racist things ordinary people said about queuejumpers and people who didn't speak English. *If you don't like it, leave.* Where did that leave me? I was only here because I was going crazy back home where I loved everything and everyone except the things that were driving me crazy. I dared not say what was most true in my heart.

In Australia, no-one seemed interested in talking politics. What was there to say about John Howard? But you could always get a conversation going about sport. It was perfectly understandable in a perfectly incomprehensible way.

It took me years before I understood the difference between Labor and Liberal. And even then, not so well.

At grocery check-outs, when asked if I had 'FlyBuys', which at first I mistook for 'fly bites', I assured the check-out girl that I most certainly did not.

Zed started to watch something called *The Footy Show*. A whole show about football, with pranks and silly jokes. I dropped my head in my hands. I didn't know if I could go on.

I wondered how to clean under the rim of a toilet and if there was a way of doing it without actually, you know, using your hands. I was ashamed I didn't know how (what sort of a person was I?) and that Violet, and then Mandisa, had always done it for me. My history was a stain that ran deep in my blood. I thought a lot about Violet and her years of indentured labour to my family, displaced from her own, thinking how she probably never had a sense of 'home' living in our backyard away from those she loved. I scrubbed our toilet, wishing just once in my life I had cleaned hers. I felt better after I got poo on my hands. (Someone told me later that it's best to wear rubber gloves, because there really is no need to get poo on your hands while cleaning the toilet.)

Mandisa wrote us a few letters that left me gutted for days, saying how much she missed the kids, how she longed to be the one to get the children ready for their first day of school and see them lose their teeth. A few months after we arrived, she wrote to tell us her husband had died suddenly.

I called her.

'Mandisa, you must get tested for HIV,' I said. I sounded like a patronising white person.

'No, it wasn't HIV,' she said. But I knew, deep in my guts, it was and I wasn't there to shake her out of her denial or take her to the doctor for anti-retrovirals. No, I was helplessly, uselessly Down Under.

In my first months in Australia, despite all the novelties, I experienced a loneliness so profound I thought I might disappear into it. This was so even with the kids flanking me, and Zed returning to me each night, wide-eyed after another day at the law firm I could see was slowly leaching his carefree spirit. My days were full of shopping, cleaning and looking after a four and two year old, whose lives and routines had been dismantled like Lego that has to go back into the box. Back in South Africa, Zed and I had been equal citizens – we both worked, earned money and raised the kids, none of this 'stay-at-home-mother' business and 'male-breadwinner' nonsense. Of course this negotiated settlement was only made possible by the peacekeeping UN presence of Mandisa.

In Australia, my world divided cleanly into the gender roles I'd worked my whole life to resist. Zed hopped on the bus for work, shaved and in a tie. I stayed at home in slippers and pimple cream with the kids. Zed got a pay cheque, I spent the grocery allowance he gave me every second Monday. Zed signed contracts for telephones and leases. I couldn't even query amenities that hadn't gone through or wonky internet connections because my name wasn't on anyone's system and I couldn't sign for anything. I choked out the words, 'Please call my partner', to verify who I was and that I had a legitimate right to query our phone bill. I was a legal minor with Zed as my guardian.

'It's just temporary,' Zed offered, the sort of fatuous consolation people idiotically offer to pregnant women about their weight.

During the day I craved adult company and to this end struck up conversations with strangers whenever I could. I thought back to all the discarded elderly people I'd seen do the same, and wondered if I'd been kind enough to them in the past. I was bitchily jealous that Zed spent all day in the city, meeting real Australians, having real conversations about torts and contracts and Starbucks' lattes over lunch. I'd make him tell me every boring detail of his day when he got home. While I was struggling with gender roles, he was just trying to get through each day, floundering to get to grips with Australian law and make sure he was providing for us. I saw the stress and responsibility in his eyes at night but I felt more sorry for me. And ever sorrier for the kids.

Jordan had tantrums by the hour. He clung to me and raged and fussed and hissed and screeched. Shannon was irritable, demanding and as rude as I'd only ever seen teenage girls. She'd left behind a singularly fantastic preschool in Cape Town that bordered on a stream and had live rabbits, tortoises and chickens running around the playground. Now here she was rightly bored hanging around with me and Jordan all day long. But I couldn't get her into a preschool, learning that in Sydney you have to book your child into daycare as soon as those two little lines on the pregnancy test pop up. I enrolled her for school in the new year but that was three long months away.

Though Jordan could only say a few words, I wondered if he missed Mandisa as much as I did in the warm peach of his heart, and what he would say to me if he could put his tantrums into words. I was certain he was uncontained because I was uncontained – he was just better at expressing his feelings. Shannon wouldn't listen to anything I said. She was moody and cross. She battled to fall asleep, so Zed and I fought every night about whose turn it was to lie with her. Everyone was running on empty.

One afternoon after a rare hour of peace and quiet, I wandered into her room to see what she was doing only to find she had drawn all over one of the walls with a permanent marker. 'Do you have any idea what they do here to people who deface rental property walls? Villawood, that's what!' I shrieked. I spent an hour scrubbing the stains with seven different types of cleaner including bleach, nail polish remover and something they call Jif, when it struck me that this was a symbolic gesture of claiming the walls as hers. Children are so poetic. I unbanned her from the naughty corner and took us all for ice-creams at the café down the road.

Sometimes we just drove around in circles listening over and over again to the story of the Little Blue Tractor. We also spent a lot of time at the play centre in Fox Studios where I drank my own body weight in cappuccinos and let the kids climb and shriek until they were broken with exhaustion.

Grocery shopping became a day's outing that had to be carefully timed between naps and after lunch to avoid arriving at the check-out with anything resembling hunger or tiredness. Dodging the Mars Bars and dinosaur lollies maliciously placed at the till became my only form of exercise. Doing the grocery shopping turned into an excursion for which I needed the whole morning to psyche myself up and from which I needed the whole week to recover. But at least it gave us something to do.

I fantasised about time on my own. Pottery. A pilates class. A quiet cup of coffee. Even wandering the aisles in the supermarket alone seemed an audacious extravagance. I wondered if I'd ever exercise or write again.

I found a spot for Jordan in daycare two days a week, then instantly regretted it. In Australia, children stay in daycare until three pm (short daycare) or six pm (long daycare). It was the longest time I'd left my children with a stranger. Though I found it self-annihilating being with the kids all day long, being apart from them was even harder. Aside from the scorching guilt, I missed the only people who needed and noticed me, and who thought I was special because I could peel the whole apple without letting the skin break.

Whenever I had a moment to myself in the day, either my five minutes alone in the shower or during a long wee, I reminded myself that loneliness accompanies all beginnings and that all beginnings are hard and all endings are sad. I wondered when the beginning would be over or whether I would forever be a beginner in this strange place.

I bought every single one of Leunig's books and put them beside my bed, a vigil against my grief.

Several weeks into this routine, Zed returned home from work and, seeing the look in my eyes, suggested I go for a walk by myself.

I fled the house and made my way down to the beach where I sat by myself as dusk crept in, looking out across the ocean, letting the sadness I had to keep under surveillance while I was with my children pool in my heart. It was getting dark, but people were about. I had never been alone on a beach at night before. I wondered if I should be scared. I looked over my shoulder. Something strange was sidling up to me, something I didn't recognise. Then it settled on me, a company as pure as the first time you see a whale leaping from the water to taste the wind. But like a handsome guy making a move, I couldn't tell if I could trust it. It took me a while to name it: it was safety. I was a safety virgin, and

I was hungry for it. I lay back in the sand and spread my arms wide to the sky, laughter stuttering from my lips. Fill me with your safety, Australia. Fuck the fear out of me. I'm all yours.

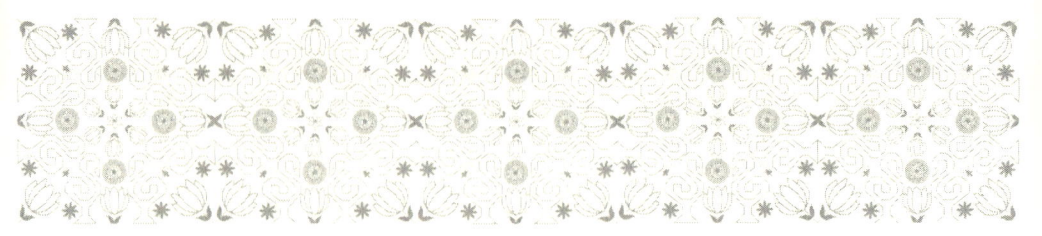

49
Zilch

Always leave a little room for a mistake.
CHINESE PROVERB

This is my fifth weigh-in with the Food Fascist and I'm feeling pretty confident. Over the past few weeks, I've dropped a couple of hundred grams every time, and once I even dropped almost a kilo.

This week, I stand on those scales and something terrible happens. These scales don't move. I haven't lost anything. Not a gram. Zilch. She doesn't say anything, just purses her lips. She can't deny it. I see her purse them.

'But I was so good . . .' I say, tears in my eyes. 'I did everything right . . .'

She doesn't reply.

'I swear, I was so good — why haven't I lost anything?'

'Take a chill pill,' she says.

Is there anything more demeaning than the patronising rhyme?

'Your body's in charge, not you,' she sniffs. 'There are a million reasons why nothing showed up today. You could be premenstrual, it could be something salty you ate so you're retaining water, you may need a big poo ... when last did you have a poo?' she asks.

I cannot tell you how uncomfortable I am discussing my bowel movements with someone who looks like a small jab might deflate her like a balloon that does a whirligig when you let it go.

'Umm, yesterday,' I say vaguely, hoping this is ample detail for her and that she's not going to ask for any kind of description.

'Are you drinking enough water?'

'Yes, eight glasses a day.'

'That's the minimum,' she says severely.

'I see,' I mumble.

'Now if you're going to get so upset by the scales, I won't let you see what they say.'

Is she talking to me like I talk to Jordan?

'Things don't always go the way we plan. We're not always in control.'

I nod miserably.

'Now, why don't you take yourself off and get a nice haircut and blow-dry. And you could do with a colour too.'

Between discussions of ablutions and beauty tips, I feel mildly bullied. Whose life is she talking about? As if I have money for hairdressing. By the time Zed and I have caught up to our peers financially, I'll have saved up enough for false teeth and a Zimmer frame. Hairdressing? Ha!

But I bite my lip.

'And next week I'm expecting a big drop, so stick to the eating plan. Use your unhappiness to be extra good this week,' she adds.

I bite my lip even harder.

Though this new eating plan has taught me a few things about restraint, I decide in this moment that I'm too grown-up to be castigated by someone else. The Food Fascist is not the boss of me. I am.

I've learned what I have to do to lose weight. I don't need the Food Fascist and her demeaning routines any longer.

'Um,' I say as I'm leaving, 'I won't be coming back next week.'

She raises her eyebrows sceptically. 'It's too soon,' she says.

And for a moment, fear tugs at me. She's right. It's too soon. I will fail if I leave now. I need her. I can't do this on my own. But this time I *recognise* fear. And, like I've been telling hunger, I tell it, '*Just be quiet, will you? No-one asked your opinion.*'

'I know what I have to do. It's just going to take time,' I say, standing my ground. 'Thanks for all your help.'

'Can you do it on your own?' she asks. 'What about support?'

I want to laugh out loud. She has no idea what I've managed to do in the past four years without any support. Has she ever had pneumonia, with two toddlers to take care of and a partner overseas, and still managed to get kids fed, bathed and into bed? She doesn't know the hours I've wept away, longing for a sister's hug or a mother's cooking to affirm my place on this earth. She knows nothing about me. But I do.

'Thanks,' I smile, liking how my voice sounds in this moment. 'But I can handle it on my own from here.'

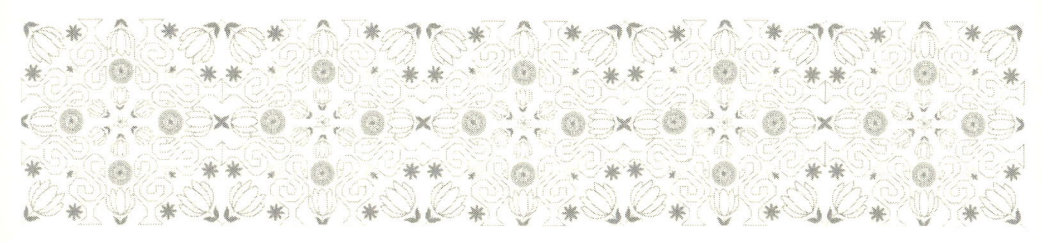

50
Small fry

Pretend you are dead and you will see who really loves you.
BAMOAN PROVERB

When I was fourteen, my pa Jack died suddenly on the operating table. My tidal grief aside (I had loved him so much), I was simply not prepared for the shock to the sensibilities that death entails. Now you see him, now you don't. Now he kisses you, now he doesn't. Now he calls you by your pet name, Josephine, now he doesn't. It's a violent assault to the mind and the body, a starvation of the senses. The absolute deprivation that is death.

I don't know about you, but death doesn't seem to get any easier for me the more people pass on. I'm as indignant and upset now when someone dies as I was when Pa did.

I don't know where the divide between breath and death is. I can't say if there's life after death or what it would feel like to be dead. I have my hopes about what happens and, if reports are to be trusted, there's a lot of white light and it isn't as scary as we imagine it to be. But we're only going to find out for sure when it actually happens to us.

No matter how we look at it, we can safely say that dying is an extinguishing of sorts. There's a space left where once a person was. People won't worry about where to seat us at a function. Someone else will have to fold the laundry if folding the laundry was our job. At the very least, our wardrobe will become redundant.

If something remains behind, a kind of negative space filled with the soul or something else ungraspable, I'll be delighted. If the dead can see the living after they pass on, fabulous. If those reports that the dead hover above those they love and protect them turn out to be true, I will certainly hover over my loved ones. Whatever it is the dead can or cannot do, I know for sure they can't cuddle the living, share a good joke or curry or call them to say, 'I've had a shocking day'. I also know that as much as people love us and imagine they cannot live without us, they really can. I'm not being cynical or hard-hearted about this. I've seen people commit to living with renewed vigour after losing their soul mates, even their beloved children. The human spirit is resilient in precisely the way we imagine it is fragile.

In our first year in Australia, I keenly felt as if *this* was the closest I'd ever come to knowing what it feels like to be dead while still breathing. For starters, I was living in a completely different time zone to the people I love. Evening here, morning there. It's the difference between two worlds. To connect at a time that's mutually convenient is like trying to line up two planets in the same orbit for a photo opportunity.

Secondly, I was physically gone. Ilze got married a few weeks after we left South Africa and I wasn't there to hear her special vows and throw rose petals. I'm sure the dead aren't nearly as miserable as I was to miss her wedding and, if celebrity psychic John Edwards is right, they're probably hovering nearby, only too pleased at having escaped the pastel bridesmaid dresses.

Without the connections of family and friends to hold me together, I felt molecularly unstable, the way ice in heat surrenders its form to a puddle and finally sighs into water vapour. It makes the soul sick to be truncated from its origin, splintered, a genetic shard. I longed for someone to push my buttons – I missed having someone know me well enough to irritate me. The people who love us don't care what we stand for, who we vote for, what our large achievements in the world are. They want to know what we ate for breakfast and if we prefer Special K with the almonds and honey or without. They know our shoe size and our colour preferences. They know we collect babushkas or owls or bookmarks or Chinese lanterns. They want to know if we've also had piles and what ointment we recommend. They'll phone us specifically to find out whether we also wet ourselves laughing at that scene in *You Don't Mess with the Zohan* when the Zohan did that thing with the hummus. We're connected to the people we love, not through Justice or Peace or Democracy or God, but through a million mundane details of everyday life that get lost; a confetti of broken intimacy when we leave.

Unmoored from these fixtures, my neat ordered life was ransacked, turned upside down and compressed like *WALL•E*'s garbage cubes. I couldn't believe my loud life had shrunk so small as I imagine the cremated must feel about their ashes. It's very difficult to envisage that this reduction is a spiritual contraction. It simply feels annihilating.

I stood in as Shannon's 'grandparent' on Grandparents' Day at school, so that she wasn't the only one sitting alone making a picture frame out of toilet rolls and pasta shells with 'Greatest

Granny in the World' written on it. I posted it back to South Africa for my mother, even though it cost a day's worth of Jordan's childcare. It arrived squashed and broken, but it was the thought that counts.

In Australia, the stories of my life, my CV, my biography, my portfolio, all I'd worked for and done, disappeared. No-one was interested in my wardrobe of glittery awards and stiletto-ed accomplishments. They were unfashionable, just wrong, the kind of thing you keep to yourself. I'd once been a big fish in a small pond. Now I was small fry. At times I felt as if I'd swallowed myself whole, history and all, and kept burping up memories.

Every day I spent hours frantically writing emails home to all my friends. To be fair, a few responded – but not with the urgency of my need, which was immediately. My family kept me going via correspondence, but what I shockingly discovered a few weeks into my emigration is that people get on with their lives without you. While people miss you, no-one's life stops because you've left. This was a dreadful realisation and I wondered if the dead take it as personally as I did. I wanted to be missed horribly. Unbearably. I wanted the vacuum I'd left in people's lives to swallow them whole. I wanted life to be not worth living ... but not really. Because I love the people I left behind, I hoped in that big-hearted way that they'd get on with their lives and do great things even if I wasn't there to share in them.

Apart from wanting to be missed by those back home, I also wanted to be noticed by the people around me. But when they did, I felt bullied. I even developed my own mini personality disorder, something verging on a persecution complex. One evening after a successful grocery shop during

Thursday late-night shopping, the woman at the check-out casually asked if she could look inside my bag.

'I beg your pardon?' I stuttered.

'Ma'am, can I please look inside your bag?

'Do you think I've *stolen* something?'

'Please just open your bag . . .' she continued.

Never in my life had anyone taken me for a thief or a cheat. As I've said before, I'm pathetically honest. I wouldn't steal a paperclip. After she'd had a cursory glance inside my handbag, I sputtered, 'See? See?'

'It's because of my South African accent,' I told Zed later that night.

This, I can now diagnose, is a neurotic narcissism in which I was the celebrity inside my own drama. Except I was a celebrity no-one recognised.

Over the weeks that followed, I noticed that just about everyone is asked to 'open their bags' for inspection at the check-out. In South Africa I'd only ever seen black people harassed in this way. *This*, then, was my first taste of real equality.

Some years later on Coogee Beach one hot Sunday afternoon, two young women sat down next to us. The blonde one was worrying that she'd grabbed her black bra instead of her black bikini top on her way out. The other assured her that 'no-one would notice'. The blonde wasn't convinced. I watched out of the corner of my eye behind my sunglasses as she got into the water – with her black bra on. Really, no-one but me noticed.

The notion that 'people are looking' is really a fiction of the ego. Most of the time, no-one is looking and no-one really cares. The idea that we matter more than we do is our little human performance, which is why men comb their remaining hair over the bald patch. As if anyone would care about a bald spot. Funnily enough, people notice the combing of the hair more than the bald spot.

As an immigrant, you must come to terms with indifference. Vast, catastrophic indifference – to your loss, your suspension, your ignorance, your unknowing, your exclusion. What is most present for you – your alienation – is both invisible and irrelevant to everyone else. You become the Sleeping Beauty in your own story, never knowing when you're going to wake up. This frozen sadness, family therapist Pauline Boss explains, happens when we cannot really know what we've lost. People who lose their loved ones to immigration, adoption, Alzheimer's or unresolved circumstances can never fully let go. The ambiguity of the loss creates confusion in the heart. It freezes the grieving process, making it difficult to detach sufficiently to achieve closure on what we've lost. An irretrievable loss, she says, is easier to mourn than one that has no clear beginning or ending.

The Zen koan asks, if a tree falls in the forest and there's no-one to hear it, does it make a sound? It's such a beautiful expression of the conundrum of unperceived existence. Can something exist if it is not perceived, or is it perception that validates existence? This puzzle continues to keep philosophers tied up in ontological knots (clearly metaphysicians don't have the big questions like stubborn stains and the cat's oozing pus-wound to worry about). In my first year in Australia, I came close to understanding what George Berkeley, an eighteenth-century Irish philosopher, meant when he said, 'To be is to be perceived.' Solitary confinement is psychological torture, precisely because human beings need to be acknowledged. Eye contact. A nod. Even a 'fuck you'. Anything.

Most painfully, the people most precious to me, my children, were invisible. It would catch me unawares, a despair so stultifying that I couldn't inhale, whenever Shannon or Jordan — my beautiful, clever, funny children — lost a tooth, cracked a joke or made an adorable 'out-of-the-mouths-of-babes' comment that clearly no other five or three year old could ever have come up with before. I'd carefully lift it up — the gesture, the comment, the swimming certificate — like an invisible broken bird, lay it gently on the cotton wool of my heart and weep into the void of 'Brilliant Things Children Do that Go Unnoticed'. I'd email my family, detailing what this one said, what that one did: 'a whole length without floaties by himself!', 'a yellow belt in karate', 'the second bottom tooth', 'he called the cat a "piece of the night"'.

One morning, after her first few months at school, Shannon was reading, PD Eastman's *Are You My Mother?* aloud. 'Time to go,' I called. She pulled her school bag onto her back and, as she passed me in the doorway, she stopped and looked me straight in the eye and said, 'I will never leave you.'

I swallowed back the reflux of my anguish, certain that we had imprinted leaving into her soul; that loss had become her emotional inheritance.

In those early days, I learned that children need to be noticed. Every inch they grow is a festival, every milestone they cross a carnival, every step they take a gala event. They need to be applauded for the effort and courage it takes to be a person. They need words like 'clever', 'well done', 'beautiful' and 'special' to be rained down on them, so that some can flow into the estuary of their spirits.

Without fans of grandparents and crowds of cousins cheering them on, they grow up anyway, because that's what children do. But they unfold like wildflowers in a desert, with nothing but the unmoved brown earth and indifferent sunlight as their witnesses.

During those first few weeks, which become months and years, I had to be careful with myself. I had to watch for self-pity, which can gather like moss at your feet, spreading its way up to your knees and then higher. Misery is a decadence you need to cut out like high-*schmaltz* snacks.

It was the smallest of things that saved me.

The six bunches of past-their-sell-by-date roses the woman at the organic fruit shop around the corner left outside my door, the ones she'd seen me admiring.

A pod of dolphins in the early morning bay that made the children squeal because they'd never seen anything so magical. *In real life.*

Someone – an Australian! – offering to pick Shannon up for school. And then noticing she'd lost a tooth.

The gym equipment which was just the same as gym equipment in South Africa – I knew how to use it without having to ask anyone for explanations or help. Except I had to sign a dozen indemnities and an adherence of 'safe gym practice'.

Questions like: 'Do you have any siblings?' 'Are your parents still alive?' *Yes, I have a family. Yes, yes, yes. Would you like to see photos?*

Emails from home helped, like the one from my friend Mmatshilo: 'Embrace the confusion, the pain, doubts and loneliness. This is called growth, Jo. It is called finding a path. Keep on asking the questions and learn to accept the answers, even if they are not the same as what you would have loved.'

In moments when I felt unsaved, I'd call home to hear the voices of those to whom I mattered, lost in their own ambiguous loss. I'd sob freely. I'd voice to my mother that I missed her – the kind of thing you never get to say to people you love when they're part of your daily life. My father would console me, 'Someday you'll be able to see this experience for what it is. In the meantime, just keep going, day by day, hour by hour. Pretend you're doing research for a book.'

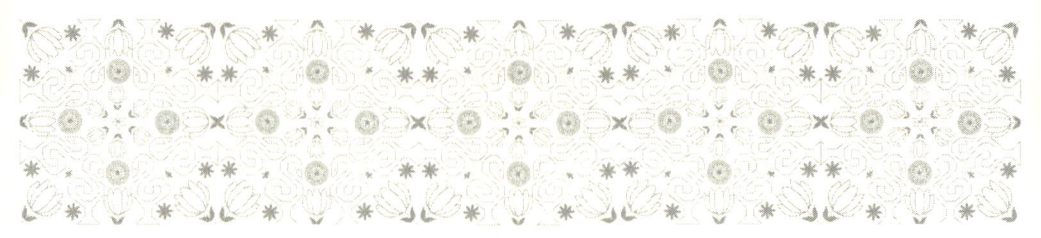

51
Snap

It is too heavy to carry and too precious to throw away.
Yiddish proverb

I'm standing in the kitchen holding a piece of plastic in one hand and a piece of metal in the other. It's probably not normal to be crying over a broken egglifter.

'Just throw it out,' Zed says.

'Can't we try to fix it?' I sob

'Just throw it away. Get another one at the two-dollar shop. They sell kitchen utensils, don't they?'

I stand over the bin for a good few minutes looking at the plastic handle, which is blue and white with yellow flowers, faded from use, but I can still make out the pattern.

This was my granny's egglifter, the very one she used to fry eggs for us when I was a little girl. It's one of the few objects I brought back from our first return trip to South Africa after eighteen months in Australia.

The last time I'd spoken to my granny I'd joked, 'Just hang on, Gran, I'll be back soon. Carry on regardless.' But she ran out of steam just weeks before we made it home.

SNAP

My granny gave me entry into a quaint old-fashioned world of beautiful manners; hand-crocheted, hot-water-bottle covers, and silverware engraved with her initials, BC. She kept china coffee sets and Spode crockery neatly dusted at the back of her sideboard. Every Saturday night, when my sisters and I slept over at her apartment as kids, she let us dress up in her clothes and jewellery of the kind I had only ever seen in movies, including large topaz rings with stones the size of small rocks. We'd wrap ourselves in her mink stoles and put on her high-heeled shoes until we outgrew her little feet. We powdered ourselves with her large powder puff and smeared on lipstick from a collection of hot pinks that smelled waxy and sweet. We played 'house' with her silverware, with angels on their handles, and filled her eggcups shaped like water lilies with Coke. She gave us liquorice, wine-gums and marshmallows as rewards for good manners. She always gave us pocket money and slipped us a sip of her whiskey on the rocks.

Despite her best efforts, she couldn't conceal that she was terrified of death. She lay awake into the wee hours of the morning listening to DJs natter on about the cricket, crime, the state of the roads, schools and the economy, worrying about how many ways there were to die and no doubt putting in her requests. The death she finally got (a necrotic stomach and perforated oesophagus compounded by a stroke) was ghastly, by death's standards. She deserved to have died as she'd lived, like a lady. 'Oh my God,' she'd have exclaimed, 'just switch off the machines.'

An ICU nurse said to Carolyn in those days, when Granny Bee was expected to die and didn't, 'They don't make people like they used to anymore.' Words my granny might have used to describe vacuum cleaners, clothes, furniture and kitchen utensils.

My granny took her last breath on the night of 8 March 2003, in a hospital bed in Johannesburg, South Africa, while I was waking in Sydney on the morning of 9 March, nine hours ahead. I had been keeping a little candle alight for her as she struggled between life and death in the sanitised surrounds of a hospital – how she hated them. For as long as I can remember, she would tell us that she 'never wanted to be a burden', and that when enough was enough, it was time to die and 'be finished with it'.

Her death so far away hurt like nothing I'd ever experienced – a referred pain, somewhere in the space between my memory and my heart. While my family gathered to bury her and say prayers, I was making up kids' lunch boxes and getting on with my daily tasks, offering unsolicited explanations to people in public for my tears: 'You see, my granny just died ...'

When that egglifter with the blue and white handle finally snapped, something in me snapped too. As it clanked its way down into the belly of the bin, I felt a little tendril sever inside.

It hurt like hell.

But I let it go. I let it go.

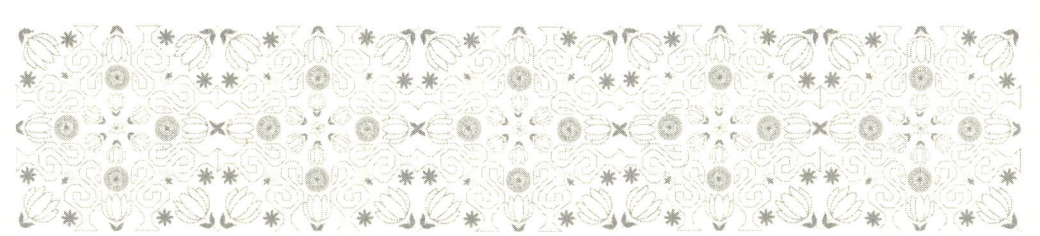

52
Seed

Before God and the bus driver, we are all equal.
GERMAN PROVERB

Granny Bee was both a horrible driver and a terrible joke teller, neither of which stopped her from getting behind a wheel or a punchline. One of her favourites, which she frequently repeated (even though I explained that once people knew the punchline, it wasn't that funny anymore), was about a man who meets a gorgeous woman on a plane. She tells him she's on her way to a nymphomaniacs' convention, to share her research that the people with the highest libidos are the Jews and the Indians. 'By the way, what's your name?' she asks. 'Hiawatha Lipschitz,' he replies.

I wish she'd stuck around long enough for me to tell her another joke, if only so she could butcher it in the retelling: two little old ladies, Ethel and Mavis, are hunched in their car seats, purple rinses bobbing above the dashboard, with Ethel at the wheel. Ethel drives through a red light and Mavis almost ladders her stockings from shock. 'Maybe Ethel's eyes aren't so good anymore. Maybe I should say something . . .' she thinks.

Knowing how her friend hates being criticised, she keeps quiet. A few minutes later, Ethel goes through yet another red light. This time Mavis really does ladder her stockings. But again, she thinks, 'Don't be a backseat driver, Mavis,' and remains silent. But when Ethel goes through a third red light, Mavis can't contain herself. 'Ethel, my dear thing,' she says. 'What's the matter with you today? You've gone through three red lights.'

'Oh,' Ethel replies. 'Am I driving?'

Personally, I prefer the driver's seat. I like to choose where to sit and to know where I'm going. But sometimes in life we're not given a choice and all we can do is be a good passenger and stop *kibitzing* from the back.

It doesn't matter where we're seated – spiritual insights come to us just as well whether we're sitting under the Bodhi tree or on the loo. Some of my most profound divine encounters have happened in the little girl's room – the sanctuary in which God let me know on two occasions I was going to be a mother.

And then there was the time, ten weeks into my pregnancy with Shannon, while I was still at Hedgebrook Womens Writers Colony, when I went to the loo and saw something that really didn't belong on the toilet paper: blood. Could it be blood? It was blood. Definitely blood. Trust me, a girl knows when there's blood. My heart roared inside my chest. *No. Please. No.* In that moment between me and the toilet paper, I was assailed by a flock of all the lonelinesses that can afflict the human spirit at once: the loneliness of being on your own, far away from people you know and love; the loneliness of being unmet in a relationship; and the singular loneliness when something isn't right in your own body, which you can't share with anyone. Because it's *your* body.

Here I was in America, far away from Zed and my family; I was surrounded by caring but indifferent strangers, and I thought I was miscarrying. I can't say I handled the situation with much personal dignity or containment, but thankfully, because I was *all alone,* there was no-one around to see me. I fell on my bed shivering and crying. I held onto my belly and I pleaded with God: *Please don't let me lose this baby.* I did yogic postures to reverse gravity. And just in case God wasn't on the case, I spoke to the baby: 'Now listen here, it's only been ten weeks, and you haven't really given me a fair chance. Please hold on . . .'

I'd wanted a baby since I was four. I'd been collecting baby clothes for years in preparation. This was so unfair. There were so many unwanted pregnancies out there. People fighting for their right to terminate. Why not miscarry those and leave me out of it? I'd always harboured reservations about God's sneaky ways – if he could tell Abraham, the forefather of the Jewish people, to sacrifice his breathing, living son, what was a little ten-week miscarriage for a nobody like me of a five-centimetre-long foetus that didn't even have toenails yet?

For several days, God played with me like I've seen Tanaka play with lizards (it never ends well for the lizard). Whenever I went to the toilet, I'd hope, *Please come up milky clean.* But there was the unmistakable blood stain. I'd wipe again, hoping this time for a different result. The same. I'd cry quietly into my hands, I suppose preparing myself for goodbye.

Spotting, as it's cutely called, a term that seems more apposite to interior decorating than obstetrics, is quite common during the first trimester of a pregnancy, so I came to learn. Some women even bleed well into their pregnancies. But without this knowledge back then, I wept myself into a floppy rag of despair. I raged against the injustice of this small mutiny in my belly.

One evening I started to wend my sorry-for-myself pregnant arse down through the trees towards the main farmhouse, where the cooks had been pottering all day in and amongst the herb gardens to cook up an organic banquet for us ravenous writers. As I reached a clearing and looked out towards the evening, which had sighed around the cathedral of Mount Rainier like a lover's breath, I paused. There was something about the bigness of that mountain against the whole tiny drama of my life and the battle for tenure going on inside my womb that gave me a moment's reprieve. It reminded me of the beautiful Buddhist parable of Kisa Gotami, who lost her only son. Desperate with grief, she brought his lifeless body to the Buddha, asking him to bring her son back to life. The Buddha agreed on condition that she bring him a handful of mustard seeds from a home in which no-one had lost a child, husband, wife or friend. Excited, Kisa Gotami set off to find the seeds, but every family whose door she knocked on had lost someone they loved. She became more and more despondent as she went from home to home, unable to find a single living person who hadn't suffered the loss of a loved one and, in the process, became enlightened in an acceptance of the impermanence of all life.

There was a strange relief in this perspective which emptied me of the sorrow, the rage, the heartbreak of my own predicament. I suddenly felt my foothold sure and firm. I wasn't being persecuted. I wasn't meant to take this personally. I put my hands over my belly and announced to the sky, 'Okay, I get it. I have no control over this. Since no-one's asked what I think, I'd just like to state that I'd prefer if this pregnancy could hold.' And then I addressed the ten-week-old foetus inside me: 'Look, I haven't been much fun over the past few days. I've been pretty wretched at the thought of losing you. I can understand if you're having doubts about coming into this world. But just in case you're unsure whether I want you, I'd like you to know that I want you more than anything. I'll do my best to hold onto you if you hold onto me. But if you change your mind, I hope you'll try again at a later stage. You see, I will try very hard to be a fantastic mother.'

With those few words, the despair and anxiety that had been weighing me down just fell away. I felt kilos lighter. As I walked down towards my delicious dinner amongst smart and funny women, I strode with a new confidence, though probably not quite enlightenment. All the lonelinesses of the past few days had left me and a comforting presence walked beside me, a silent hand in mine.

And in that moment, when I let go and stopped trying to control things, I made space for God.

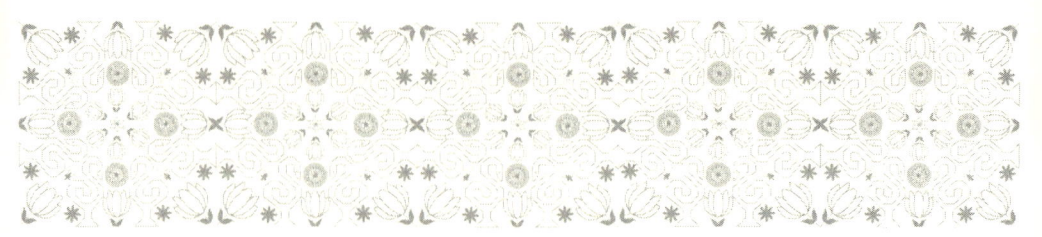

53
Rite

The tears running down your face do not blind you.
TOGOLESE PROVERB

Were penises a matter of preference, and not part and parcel of a delightful but fairly inflexible marital set-up, in a choice between circumcised and uncircumcised I'd always pick circumcised. I can only attribute this irrational preference to my tribal heritage, which insists on the early removal of the foreskin. Women are excused from witnessing the nitty-gritty of ritual Jewish circumcision, but in my early teens my curiosity got the better of me and I found myself standing within arm's reach of the *mohel* (the rabbi who does the circumcision). And let me just say: 'Eeeuw.' Despite claims to the contrary to placate anxious mothers of newborns, I can't believe it doesn't hurt.

If you've ever inadvertently sliced your finger while wielding a very sharp knife, you'll appreciate that what's really going on during a circumcision is carvery. This is the job of a butcher or a surgeon. There's really no getting away from the fact that scalpel will pierce flesh. Notwithstanding this surgical reality, an odd vaudevillian sense of gaiety accompanies this ritual, and no sooner has the little fella had his johnson trimmed and is rightly wailing his head off than everyone is scoffing back chopped herring with an air of bewildering festivity.

When it came time for Jordan to be circumcised, I burrowed myself in the room furthest away from the proceedings, blubbing whenever I heard his squeaks and squawks and finally bellow of protest. I had to employ every ounce of self-restraint not to break up the party and snatch my son away before the blade touched his winky.

I'm grateful I don't belong to a tribe that slices girls' clitorises off, knocks front teeth out or chucks you out in the wilderness for a week to see if you can survive. Because life would be truly miserable without a clitoris or front teeth, and I'd put money on me getting lost in the wilderness without a map. But many cultures employ some form of ritual to mark a milestone or to put initiates on trial to prove they're worthy of tribal membership.

The word 'initiation' derives from the Latin word for 'entrance' or 'beginning' and, as such, is a spiritual doorway into a new existential state and deeper tribal consciousness where the sacred is revealed and spiritual values are passed on. It marks the loss of spiritual virginity (farewell to the hymen of innocence) and the acceptance of new awareness and responsibilities. Anthropologically, initiation is regarded as a spiritual death, and a rebirth into a new consciousness.

If one is going to be initiated I reckon it's best not to know what's coming, to avoid panic at the pain that is certainly on its way and, more spiritually, perhaps to facilitate Beginner's Mind. So I've come to this modest understanding: the very essence of initiation is that it *is* bewildering, that it must be undergone dumbly and blindly. It's not a choice we make, but an imposition to which we yield. We succumb to it for reasons that are not clear to us and, in submitting, we are 'shepherded' by the older generation, other tribal members (or perhaps God) through a portal. When (and *if* in some cases – a few of those circumcisions get yuckily infected) the test is passed, we're rewarded with deliverance in a sensation perhaps no more gratifying, edifying or enlarging than that of having survived.

Initiation is a 'baptism by fire', a term describing a soldier's first experience of battle (from the French *baptême du feu*, derived from the ancient Greek *baptisma pyros*). Despite its sophisticated European lineage, it seems to me to be just be a fancy way of saying, 'Thank God that fucking nightmare is over'.

When I was in high school my geography teacher disappeared for a whole semester, rumoured to have suffered a 'nervous breakdown', a term that to this day conjures up images of skinny Mrs Beden convulsing in a heap of dressing gowns and curlers, streaked with tears of mascara, spooning ice-cream into her mouth from a five-litre tub. I've always quietly wondered what it was that had finally thrown her down the stairwell of her life, and if it was something big like the death of a friend, or something little like a parking fine.

Two weeks after our arrival in Sydney I contemplated whether perhaps Australia would be the catalyst for my own nervous breakdown. Early motherhood taught me that postnatal depression isn't fussy in the least. It's a wanton Casanova and will indiscriminately mount competent and well-adjusted women who themselves were breastfed as babies and brought up in loving homes. In Australia, I experienced a type of post-traumatic stress brought on by the desertion of all my accumulated competencies (and what a competent girl I was used to being). I was irrationally brought to tears over the smallest thing. Let's see: I'd cry every time we heard eighties band Toto on the radio blessing the rains down in Africa. I'd cry (in public) when we'd arrive too late for the library story-time which only had twenty places and which were already taken. I'd cry when other South Africans invited us for Shabbat dinner, and I'd cry when no-one invited us for dinner. I cried during adverts, especially with puppies and babies. I cried as if there was nothing between other people's pain and my own.

Really, without wanting to sound too much like a basket case, I considered that in a choice between my anxiety-fuelled insanity in South Africa and my bawling incompetence in Australia, I'd have preferred to have remained with Mandisa and Table Mountain and made inquiries about a good psychiatrist.

The only sobering rampart to this self-erosion was some tentative awareness that I should try to not let the children see me cry. I couldn't always offer Shannon a rational response to her legitimate and recurring inquiry, 'Why are you crying?' Jordan, who always woke up from his afternoon nap crying, would need to be held in my arms for half an hour, where I'd coo, 'It's okay, my baby, it's okay,' until he calmed down and realised that actually it wasn't so bad to be awake. It bothered me, it bothered me a great deal when he waddled over to me one day, cocked his head and patted my hair saying, 'It's okay, my baby.'

In the movies, when someone is on the run or is altering identities, there's often that scene in front of the mirror in which they wildly cut their hair. As someone who spent years growing my own, I know that no-one just chops off chunks of hair. You have to be desperate.

My granny loved my hair. When I was a little girl, she used to brush it for me until it shone like 'a silken curtain'. I was born with a mop of black hair like a bottlebrush, and probably have more than anyone really needs. I've worn it long my whole life, tangling necklaces and the odd man in it. When I breastfed Shannon, she found a strand to play with, twirling it round and round her little fingers until she fell asleep.

Just before we left South Africa, my hair had finally grown to cover my nipples. It was a vanity that had taken years. After just a few short weeks in Australia, something happened with my hair. It got knotty at the back with little dreadlocks. On the beach, the wind slapped it in my face. Each time I tied it back I did so more and more tightly.

After six months of this hair unhappiness, I stood in front of the mirror in the bathroom and, with a pair of blunt children's paper scissors, I cut off huge chunks. The dark locks fell and scattered onto the white tiles of the bathroom floor, years and years of patient growth now just a fluff of fallen follicles.

I didn't notice her at first, but then I saw Shannon standing in the doorway, tears running down her face.

'Don't do that, Mommy. I like you with long hair,' she sobbed. 'You don't look like my mommy anymore.'

'*Mummy*,' I said. 'Here they say *mummy*.'

Looking back now, I see that our first three years in Australia were a taxing and lengthy initiation without any of the spiritual equanimity you'd hope might illuminate such experiences. Here's some idea of how those years clocked up: Zed was away on business in Kuala Lumpur when a dreadful exhaustion accompanied by a pain in my chest was confirmed as pneumonia. I spent six weeks in bed, coughing. While coughing, I put my back out (taking the concept of a *rachmonis* to a whole new level).

Just as my pneumonia and back were starting to settle, Zed, following our equable agreement that we should each do things we enjoy lest we end up slowly marinating in our loathing of one another, joined an indoor soccer team and ruptured his Achilles tendon in the first game. He then spent the next three months on crutches. During this time he was retrenched due to the world financial crisis post-9/11. We had three months left on our temporary visa for him to find another job or else we had to go home. By this point, South Africa seemed like a paradise and I couldn't wait to get back. It was pretty clear Australia just wasn't all that into us.

'Let's get the hell out of here and go back home,' I said to Zed.

Zed pointed out that we'd spent a lot of time, energy and money to get to Australia and perhaps we should try to stick it out and get citizenship for the kids. 'At least that way, they'll have choices. We can always go back home after that.'

He is infuriatingly sensible.

Over the next two months, Zed applied for over seventy jobs and was called back for interviews for three. We had *ten* days left on our temporary visas when he was offered a new job at a fraction of the salary of the job that had brought us to Australia. At this point, even baked beans on toast looked like a hideously extravagant luxury.

Christians, I'm sorry to say, have got one thing wrong. Hell is not the worst place. For starters, hell is a location. It has an address. You can unpack your suitcase in hell, you can knock as many nails as you desire in the walls of purgatory. You can plant your autumn bulbs in the valley of brimstone. No, the worst place to be is neither here nor there. A limbo. Always looking back. Never fully present in the moment. Frozen between your past and present. During those early years in Australia, I always felt that at any moment I might spiral away, without the gravity of my own sense of place to hold me to the earth.

I put my head down and tried to just get through each day with a little less hurt at the fact that the phone never rang, that I never dressed right for the weather, that in my dreams I was always lost, rummaging.

My friend Brandon, whom I'd known since we were student activists together at university fighting for a new future for South Africa, sent me an email during this time saying: 'We need you. We love you. We miss you. You belong to us. Come back home.'

And I feasted on those words 'need', 'love', 'miss', 'belong' and 'home', like a starveling.

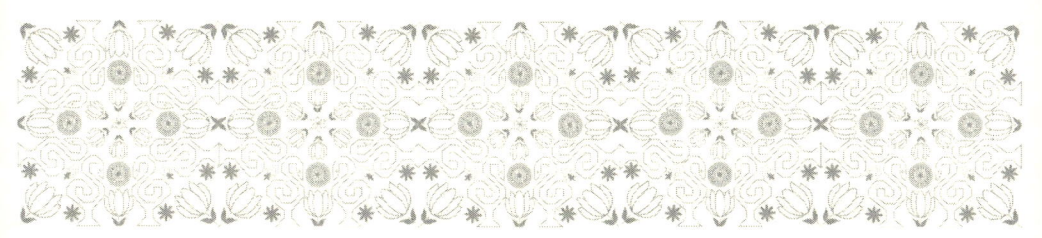

54
Eyeball

Only through the eyes of others can we really see our own faults.
CHINESE PROVERB

I'm dropping my friend Jane's son off when she leans in at the window of my car. She pauses and squints at me.

'You look different. Have you lost weight? Your face seems thinner,' she says, giving me the eyeball.

My face? Of all the places I need to lose weight, my face is last. A skinny face only enhances the size of my nose. I don't need a size 8 face. I mean, what will that bully Rufus Kremansky have to say?

But in this moment, something in me billows. My heart soars. *Someone has noticed!* There is change, incremental as it may be. My chin is pointier, my cheeks more hollow. It's happening, slowly. I smile my biggest smile and I say, 'Yes, I've lost three and a half kilos. Thanks for noticing.'

I've been on this new eating plan for nine weeks now and I'm feeling pretty darn good. There is a little lilt in my three-and-a-half-kilo lighter step. I walk with my head held higher. I'm even thinking of having my big nose pierced – I've wanted to for ages, but was always too scared, because what would people say? But I remember something from when I backpacked through Malawi with Max and we met a young boy called Binos who took us on a dugout to a paradisiacal island where we snorkelled and ate mangos the size of rugby balls. On the dugout, a hollowed out tree trunk which forms a curved boat, were engraved the words 'Let Them Say'. I asked Binos what the name meant and he explained that in Malawi, which is one of the poorest countries in Africa, in order to own a dugout you need to buy a tree from the government. To buy a tree costs a lot of money. When you buy a tree, people will say, 'That is a rich man – he has a lot of money.' Let them say.

These days I'm not so attached to what other people think or say about me.

I've learned to order my coffee lean and mean – without the baggage of a muffin or banana bread. I mean, who're they kidding? They're both cake in disguise and I know better now. My pants are ever so much looser on me. Unfortunately, so are my bras – a fact Zed has taken to lamenting. But – and of course, he'll deny this – his libido seems to have stepped up a notch, which is as necessary as another facelift for Joan Rivers. I can't tell whether he's been lying all along about finding me sexy while secretly harbouring a desire for a skinnier me all these years, or whether it's my own sexual appetite which has displaced my gastronomic one that has plumped his. But three and a half kilos down, I definitely feel more erection-worthy.

I haven't been back to the Food Fascist, but I have stuck to my new eating plan. All by myself. Day by day, meal by meal, mouthful by mouthful, I'm becoming aware of a new power. It's the slow accrual of consciousness, laid down like sheaths of mother-of-pearl, that despite all the things in the world over which I have no control – like the rising price of petrol and mortgage rates, the little wrinkles that are appearing around my eyes when I smile, the crash of the stock markets, the health and wellbeing of the people I love, what people think of me or whether they even do, whether cancer will strike now or later – there is one thing over which I do have control.

I'm in control of everything I choose to put in my mouth.

Sometimes in life, we are Mavis. And sometimes we are Ethel. And it's important to know the difference.

When eating, *I* am driving.

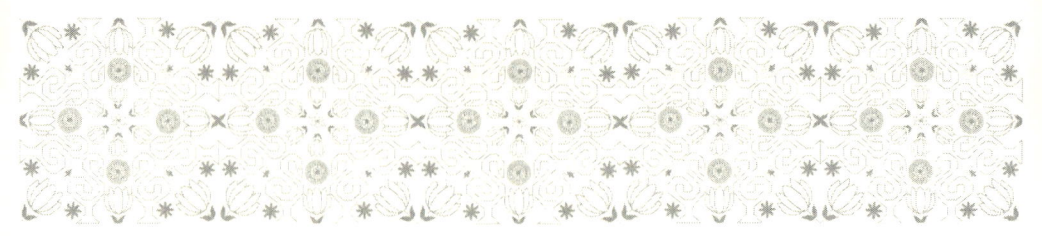

55
Rearview

The sickness of the body is the cure of the mind.
BASQUE PROVERB

With the 10,000 steps I've been doing religiously every day, which has involved some running and stair-climbing, my hamstrings have clammed up, making me hobble when I walk, which isn't such a good look, even for the svelte. It's astonishing how much unsolicited advice people are willing to dispense in the face of a limp, but it all boils down to one word: yoga. The exercise of the gods, yoga, by all accounts, makes you younger and stronger and it's also good therapy for sulking hamstrings. I actually did yoga all through my childhood while my parents were going through an Eastern phase. My father even had a yoga guru before he became *Lubavitch*.

So I join a yoga studio in Bondi full of obscenely beautiful and supple people who fluently tie the sculpture of their bodies into a ribbon of limbs. We get to hum and chant and lie quietly and still call this exercise. For weeks, I am calm and centred and can reach my toes. But then – can one stomach the irony? – I *over*stretch (I must be the world's only yoga over-achiever) and put my back out. I mean, really.

For the next two weeks, I have to lie flat on my bed with a rolled-up towel under my knees, forced to remember a man from my past who wanted to shag me which, at the time, seemed like a decent compromise to love. He was very sexy and smart and so I wanted to shag him back. During an adventurous shagging marathon, performed with various acrobatics I was probably not equipped to handle, I acquired a prolapsed disc. I believe I actually heard that disc groan. Since then I've carried the lingering memory of this racy and tempestuous love affair, most particularly when I don't bend properly or I carry something too heavy.

Putting one's back out, while grammatically similar, is a world apart from putting the garbage out. It's a grotesque euphemism for agonising and debilitating pain, combined with the inability to move one's body (not even from one side of the bed to the other). When I have to rely on others to pull up my underwear after a wee, I think to myself that though my lover was sexy 'n' all, I'd like to punch him in the balls.

Since then, I've treated my back like a toddler prone to a tantrum at any time. I try not to provoke it. But it can still erupt unexpectedly, even, you'll notice, when I do something nice for it. I am, as a result, not as fond of my back as I would like to be. I wish it would grow out of its unpredictable moods and just start behaving like a grown-up back.

My friend Kaaren sympathetically suggests I go see her body therapist, who has done wonders for her bad neck.

The body therapist is barefoot with well-looked-after toes and smells of tea-tree oil. She tells me that 'the issues are in the tissues', and that the body is a system of unsurpassable intelligence. We carry our histories, our memories, our shames and our pains in its cells. Perhaps, she suggests, my back is trying to 'tell me something'. She then asks me how I would describe my body if I were to use a metaphor.

A hippopotamus? No, not anymore. I don't think hippos can feel their hipbones. A tree? I don't feel that grand, or that grounded. Finally I say, 'A vase, that's been broken and put back together. It's got a crack all the way down.'

'Can you remember a time when you felt differently about your body, when it was whole?'

I have to trawl a long way back through my history, but yes — yes, come to think of it, I can.

Though I'm generally not a fan of photos of myself, there's one I like that was taken in Malawi with Max. Granted it was after four weeks of living on those luscious mangos and little else, and carrying a twenty-five kilo pack on my back, day in and day out. I'm walking with my back to the camera, wearing nothing but a very short sarong around my waist and a bikini top. In this photograph my back is muscled and strong. If it's permissible to say this about oneself, it is quite a sexy back. Max, who took this picture, once insisted that my back was the sexiest part of my body (which is like telling the fat girl she has a lovely personality). Too bad I'd never actually seen my back. Looking at that photo in Malawi, I can see his point.

As I begin to stitch the connections between my heart and my body, my back and my food, something Thanissara once said at a meditation retreat comes swinging back to me on the vines of obscured memory: 'Each thing has the ability to wake us up if we are there to meet it, if there is nothing in the way of it.'

REARVIEW

My back, much as it has caused me some of the worst physical pain I have endured in my life, has taught me three lessons:

1. Sometimes the best parts of ourselves are the parts we cannot see.
2. The best and most beautiful parts of ourselves are sometimes also the weakest parts.
3. To live in that magical space of incongruities is to inhabit a wormhole of real truth.

It takes me some time. I have to rummage through a lot of old boxes but I find my photographs eventually. I flick through decades of friends and misadventures and face-painting parties and baby pictures. And there it is.

I replace the picture on the fridge with the one from Malawi.

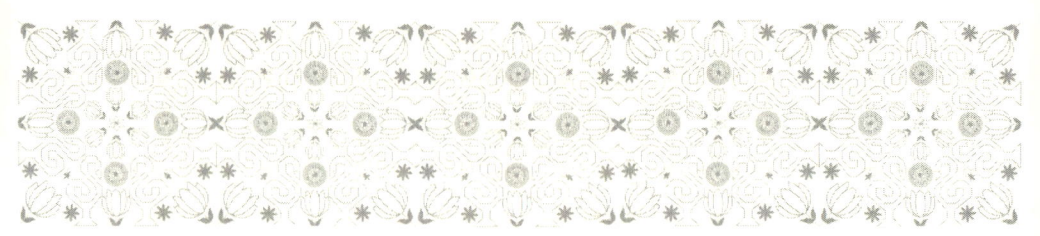

56
Chop wood

The cure for bad times is patience.
ARABIAN PROVERB

My *zaide* once told my father, 'You will do for me a picture from the Peretz story. It will be of the rabbi at the *pripetshok* [fireplace] making a fire. Behind will be the old lady on the bed. You will make the young man peering around the door.'

This was, you understand, his way of asking nicely. My dad obliged and painted this picture for his father according to his specifications where it hung in his home as his greatest pride and joy. I remember the painting well. The Isaac Leib Peretz short story 'If not higher' tells of a rabbi who would mysteriously disappear on the night before Rosh Hashana (Jewish New Year) yet no-one knew where he went. Word on the street was that he'd go up to heaven to open the gates so that the prayers of his congregation would be heard by the Almighty. A curious young fellow followed him one night, watching as the rabbi took off his holy garments and put on the clothes of a peasant, grabbed an axe and marched off into the forest. There he spent hours chopping firewood before making his way through the forest to a forsaken cottage in which a sick old woman lay in icy cold. The rabbi then lit a fire, made the old woman some soup and porridge and left. The following day in synagogue, when the congregation was speculating that the rabbi had been to heaven the night before, the young man simply responded, 'If not higher'.

My *zaide*, being a practical man, loved this story. Cleanliness? That was for fancy people. Godliness was to be found in getting your hands dirty. To *Zaide*, no person nor job was beneath him. Had he been born in the East, his philosophy could've been summed up in the Zen axiom: 'Before enlightenment, chop wood, carry water; after enlightenment, chop wood, carry water.' For those of us hoping for a post-epiphany lifestyle change, this could come as something of a letdown.

A quick glance through history, though, reveals that the greatest mystics and spiritual leaders have led lives of disarming humility – Jesus started off in a manger, Buddha sat under a tree, and Ghandi and Mother Theresa wore rags. Einstein, too, once said that if he had not become one of the world's greatest scientists, 'I think I would have enjoyed being a plumber', for which apparently the Plumbers and Steamfitters Union in Washington DC granted him an honorary membership and a New York plumbers' local presented him with a gold-plated set of plumber's tools.

Humility comes from the Latin *humus*, or 'earth', which explains why the meek are destined to inherit the earth rather than those preening on the red carpet. Humility, widely regarded as one of the greatest spiritual qualities, tempers the ego. It reins in self-importance so we don't take ourselves too seriously or things too personally – whether failure or success.

Humility is to the soul what perspective is to the eye. Far from making us smaller, humility enlarges us.

When you come from privilege, as I do as a white South African, and you arrive in a place where you have to chop your own wood, carry your own water and clean your own toilets, you quickly realise that other people have been doing your dirty work for a long time and you didn't even know it. There is, you discover, a world of difference between passing your own water and actually carrying it.

So many details of our early years of immigration would be lost if I hadn't documented them in my journals – the daily traumas, the minor indignities, the bewildering interactions, which themselves became a new sheaf of history. For as much as human beings are consumed with remembering, we are notoriously good at forgetting.

I have had plenty of time to mull over the phrase 'time heals all wounds', though people who dole out such slick platitudes generally need a good slap. It's not a generous offering to someone who is in deep pain. Grief is a consuming business and, like early motherhood, it lacks the very salvation to make it endurable, namely the big picture. But no matter whether you're serving a prison sentence, expecting a baby, or trying to lose weight, time will pass. It's one of those absolutely reliable rudiments of human existence.

For what seemed like a very long time in Australia, I was painfully unsure. My default mode was disorientation, a hesitation of the footstep. I vacillated in my bearing in all manner of things. I lost all self-confidence. I was grotesquely homesick, that plague of the spirit for which there are no vitamins or antidotes. Untreated, it can easily lead to the kind of depression from which Tennyson's Mariana suffered. For ages, I felt as if I had a slow leak somewhere, and didn't know where it was or how to plug it, but I think this is what is meant by 'pining'. It's a fixation on absence. I pined for Highveld thunderstorms, the cawing of hadidahs, *Egoli* (a South African soap opera), the slang spoken on streets – things I'd never imagined were in the running for things to be missed.

All I wanted was to feel 'at home', even though I didn't myself understand exactly what I meant by this. It wasn't about real estate so much about place, something between earth and sunlight. It was about the table and sharing bread, and occasions for happiness with people who cared about the same things that trouble me. It was about losing inhibitions and finding things funny. Home is as deep as the lullaby in our blood that was sung to us when we were lulled to sleep as children, which can never be sung out. And sometimes in a birdcall that echoes of the 'Kwehh' of the Grey Lourie, or the smell of corn we grew up with as 'mielies' carried on the heads of mielie ladies, or the taste of something verging on chutney or dry 'wors' (sausage), we hear its music, a fragmented melody in the ice-cream truck of our hearts.

Home is the anthem in the bones. It's the nostalgia of our creation, a long, slow, aching hunger.

You try different things. Nothing you feed it suffices. Eventually you surrender. *Thy will be done.*

You learn to live with the emptiness. Meanwhile, you chop wood. You carry water.

The only sensible suggestion I can offer anyone from my own experience of immigration is not to determine the future of a relationship based on the first few years of a major change. You may well detest the person you most love and depend on during that time. These feelings have nothing to do with that person, nor are they a reliable gauge of the sustainability of your connection. They are the fallout of our human clumsiness; evidence of the way in which we take out our frustrations on the very people who are keeping us going emotionally, psychologically and spiritually.

There were many times when I couldn't imagine Zed and I would survive as a couple. I unconsciously blamed him for my loneliness and heartache. I was as out of touch with my own behaviour as it is possible to be, thrashing around like a fish on the sand, whacking whatever was in my path, mostly Zed (sorry, Babe).

We fought about the toilet roll. And the kind of toilet paper I bought. Why couldn't it be plain? Why did it have to be the scented kind that smelt like some Parisian brothel, not that he'd ever been in one? We fought about the mess. Mine and the kids. We fought about what took me so long to get ready and the phone bill. We fought about arrangements. There were too many on the weekends. He just wanted to relax. I just wanted company. *Then you go. Fine, I will.* So I did. Without him but with the kids. We fought about the way we spoke to each other. The tone. Was it necessary?

But he always said 'goodbye' before he left in the mornings. And 'I love you'. Just in case. I didn't always say it back.

Zed blamed me for being such a whiney pain in the arse. And who can blame him? I really was. I was the least lovely Joanne imaginable. We bickered, we sniped, we could not muster compassion for one another; we were like two blind fencers, jabbing wildly. The rainfall of all the goodness and gentleness between us drained out hopelessly to sea, instead of into the catchment of our togetherness. I often considered the tragic prospect that the only tangible outcome of our immigration might be a split. Once Zed said, in an anguish I've seldom seen him display, 'What happened to the woman I fell in love with?' I didn't know myself.

In the meantime, I counted pennies for a coffee, found excuses to go out when Zed was home at last, and wore pyjamas all day long in our rental in the suburbs, appraising the laundry as if it all just might come to life and fold itself. I checked the email every few minutes as if – oh, I don't know – someone might remember me. I was a *rachmonis* of the worst kind.

Zed and I both dreaded Friday nights. Zed because he knew I was going to be horrible company as I souped in my sadness. I, because around a Shabbat table, our little family of four seemed pathetic, denuded. To fill up the empty places, I began to invite other new immigrants for Shabbat. The Kahns, more and more often. Sometimes we were invited to join others around their tables. I noticed how sad others became over Jewish holidays and Shabbats and anniversaries and birthdays. I began to appreciate how much our presence was a bulwark for them and how much their presence shored up our losses. We knitted closer to others in a surrogacy of affection.

We dreamed about owning a home someday, but the Sydney property market is a millionaire's playground. I wondered – but only on days when my EFTPOS transaction was 'denied' and I had to leave the groceries behind – if we'd made a mistake saying no to the money back in South Africa.

'We'll never be able to afford to buy a house here,' Zed sighed, looking through the *Sydney Morning Herald* property section one morning. I kept the unruliness of a longing for a home of our own packed away, like the pictures we couldn't hang up. We watched with courteous envy as friends 'renovated', a concept as removed from our reality as vacations to Tahiti. In Sydney there seemed to be an endless hunger for property and 'home improvement', with reality TV shows dedicated to this hankering.

Meanwhile, in rented spaces made homely with our African belongings, we made our way through time. The kids started school and learned how to swim, cycle and boogie-board. They made friends. Time passed in the most ordinary way.

Bad shit happened too. We were burgled and our radios, jewellery and my laptop were stolen. After Zed's retrenchment we had to move to a more affordable suburb (actually, I moved us – with Zed on crutches he couldn't even pack his own things). Our landlord, a grumpy old man with a walnut for a heart, refused to fix things that broke in his run-down rental property, unable to be shaken from his delusion that anything that needed fixing had obviously been broken by us. He refused to send a plumber to deal with the sewage that leaked intermittently along our driveway, accusing me of flushing tampons down the toilet. Not once in my life have I ever flushed a tampon down the toilet, though I fantasised about flushing him down the toilet.

After Zed was retrenched, we could no longer afford Shannon's private school so we moved her into a public school.

When Tanaka got bitten by another cat and had a seeping wound that would cost $500 to drain, I put on gloves and I squeezed it myself.

We couldn't afford a cleaner so I cleaned. Sort of. And always with rubber gloves.

We couldn't afford babysitters so we played a lot of board games with the kids. I started to excel at UNO. Sometimes we had a night out on the town at Hungry Jacks where you could get four burgers plus bottomless drinks for under twenty dollars. The children filled up on carbonated soda till their eyes watered.

Zed – after his Achilles was healed, and had recovered from a bout of chickenpox – rode his bike to work to save on petrol.

Gym membership I'd taken for granted in South Africa was a ridiculous extravagance. Instead, I walked from Bronte to Bondi in the fresh air.

For my sisters' birthdays, I bought beads and made necklaces for them which I posted back to South Africa. The mindless creativity of beading held me steady, one bead at a time, with something lovely to show for my time. I started making necklaces to pass the days. Some kind people even bought them. In this way I kept up a small but steady income for a year making jewellery.

When all the things we could no longer have were out of our grasp, I reached down inside myself and came up with something else, something that didn't always feed the hunger, but sufficed. Made do.

Losing your home – whether voluntarily or involuntarily – is the death of the ego. This isn't so terrible when you understand that the ego is the spoilt brat of the human personality. It will do anything to be noticed, and throws a hissy fit to draw attention to itself. The higher self is that wise old sage of the human personality, not talking much, taking everything in with a sense of humour about it all.

'Look at me, look at me,' the ego whines.

'Let it be, let it be,' the higher self soothes.

When the ego has been annihilated, and all the attachments of one's self have been peeled away, what happens? Do we disappear? Actually, something else occurs: new space opens up. It's the emptiness made possible by hunger, a place from which to start afresh.

I don't know when I stopped feeling sorry for myself, but every now and then I looked in the mirror and saw someone new emerging, a whole treasure of secret selves that resourcefulness was birthing, the kind of self that, in my granny's words, 'carried on regardless'.

I stopped saying 'I can't' and just did what had to be done. I like to think I developed some humility in the process.

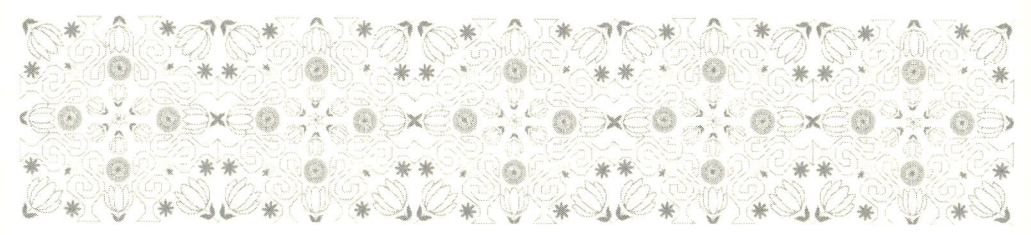

57
Training

Wisdom travels by oxen.
YIDDISH PROVERB

Zed is lying on the bed patting the spot beside him, saying, 'Jump, Tanaka, jump!'

Tanaka licks her paws and looks up at him, bored.

'Jump, Tanaka. I know you can do it, jump!'

She blinks.

'Go on, Tanaka, jump!' he urges.

And as if she has nothing better to do, she does, jumping clear of his stomach and landing on the other side with a meowful yelp.

'Good girl,' he says, stroking her head. 'Now jump the other way,' he says patting the spot she's just jumped from.

She turns around, flicking her tail in his face and, without further ado, she jumps again.

If I didn't have 3700 more steps on my pedometer to do, I would stand and watch him continue his little tête-à-tête with Tanaka, for she will keep this up as long as she's not distracted by crippling jealousy, rampant vanity or a moment of illuminated self-consciousness.

In a bout of insomnia, Zed has trained Tanaka to jump. Cats, have you noticed, are particularly difficult to train, contemptuous as they are of instructions and notoriously hard to woo with affection. But this is not Zed's first trained cat. While I was at Hedgebrook all those years ago, he taught my cat Rain to 'fetch'. This trick involved a scrunched up piece of paper which Zed threw and Rain collected in her mouth and returned to him. The modesty of this antic in no way attests to the hundreds of hours Zed must have spent training Rain, who was not the sharpest slinky on the block.

I've considered that perhaps Zed is, unbeknownst to him, a cat whisperer. Perhaps it also goes to show that with enough patience, dedication and the absence of your lover to fill your lonely nights, you could train a cockroach to sing 'La Boheme'.

The Guinness Book of Records is filled with a dizzying assortment of human beings who have, out of boredom, psychosis or insomnia, trained themselves to do a bizarre range of feats, from chewing glass to feeding their bodies through a stringless tennis racquet or collapsing their entire bodies into a small perspex box.

Training is a process that accrues by increments, as anyone who has learned a musical instrument or run a marathon knows. No-one wakes up one day and is able to fold themselves into a tiny box. No, it begins with a quirky aspiration, a 'what if?' It progresses with putting one's foot behind one's head. It goes on to an attempt to do the same with the other foot. Then it is perhaps connected by one's elbows joining the party. And so on and so on until one day you're able to put it all together seamlessly and impress passers-by by squashing yourself into a small glass cube, in the hope that they will be sufficiently impressed to leave a couple of coins in your hat.

On a recent meditation retreat, I was reminded how much I hate sitting still for lengthy periods on those little stools or cushions. My right leg always gets pins and needles. My knees hurt. The tops of my feet burn. My neck and shoulders ache. But I also remember that when I started meditating I couldn't sit for longer than five minutes without needing to move. Over the years, as I've sat in meditation, I have trained myself to ignore the pains in my legs and my back and my numb leg, knowing that it's nothing more than a niggle, that nothing will 'happen' if I don't move. My leg won't go from numb to gangrenous to having to be amputated. The irritation will pass. Eventually.

These days I can sit still for up to half an hour without needing to move. I don't think I'm less uncomfortable, just that I'm more patient with my discomfort.

It's this patience I'm learning when it comes to eating. I'm training myself to be more comfortable with my hunger. No-one can just wake up one day and be able to eat less. There will be long hours of practice that will have to precede that. Some days are easier than others. Sometimes we lose the thread and overeat. Some days we are steady. But eventually, over time, with a history of bad days and good days clocked up, it gets easier. Every day in which I get a little more at ease with hunger, I advance. Discipline is a patience with the self as I learn the new trick of eating when hungry. All spiritual practice incorporates the three elements of awareness, intention and repetition. When you repeat an action, with mindfulness and purpose, you shape a pattern, cut a groove. Coming back to the same place more than once is how you create history.

This is training.

Part Five

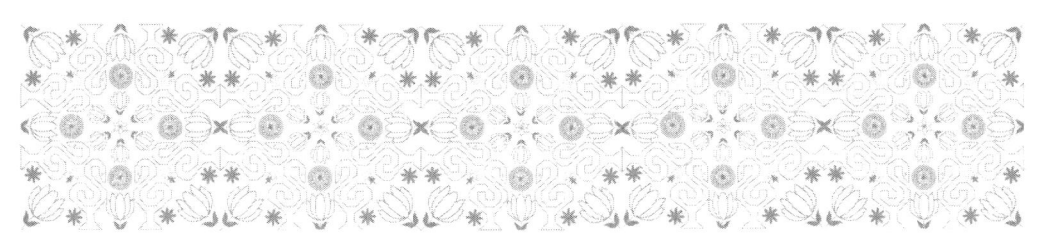

Home

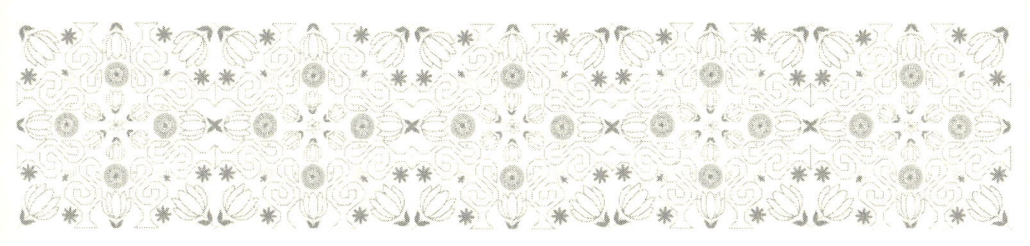

58
Return

It is often more difficult to come back home than it is to go away.
CHINESE PROVERB

The first time you go home is like bumping into an ex you haven't seen in ages, and have only just managed to get over, whom you end up sleeping with. Though you'll kick yourself for it later, your resolve will melt, all your hard work will be undone, your wounds will be re-opened as you wonder why you left him after all – he was so lovely and did that special thing with his tongue. He just has to look at you and you're a goner.

Back in South Africa for the first time after eighteen months in Australia, I was a goner. My heart got caught on the thorns of familiar things, the bird calls, the African women carrying their parcels on their heads, the over-crowded taxis culling the South African population, the warmth of its people. Australia is a lover with a slow gentle hand who won't take advantage of you. But Africa is that bad boy you'll never stop wanting who'll always have a hold over you.

South Africa's easy familiarity teased me, the way it knew me so well, all the things I love and detest. I knew all its secrets. I wondered if it might take me back. I couldn't pass a street vendor without emptying my wallet and buying beaded key rings and wire objects to take back to show my Australian friends the riches of my home. Zed worried Australian customs might take this as an attempt to start a small business in African curios. I drove past every house I'd ever lived in, rang the doorbells and peered through the barbed wire, feasting on my past. I took Shannon and Jordan to the zoo, and to the Emmarentia Dam where I bored them with stories of how I used to sunbake with my friend Stephanie when we both had crushes on the same guy who used to row there.

Returning to the embrace of my family, I watched as the kids plumped like raisins in water with all the love and attention. Shannon and Jordan became suspended in the amniotic plasma of emotional scrutiny and robust adoration. The balloon of my responsibility for them momentarily lightened, blessed with the helium of kinship.

Back home I was fed with the food of my mother's hand, made fat at her ladle. I bumped into teachers from my past, the mothers of old school friends and ex-boyfriends in shopping malls. 'Are these your children? Aren't they gorgeous?' People to whom I'm no stranger, and to whom my children are worthy of close observation. 'He has your eyes.' 'That hair – it's just like yours!'

I'd missed my granny's funeral by weeks, so my mother fast-tracked the unveiling of her tombstone so I could be there. I stood at her grave and cried all by myself – everyone else had already cried their tears of farewell, but I was emotionally jetlagged.

We then packed away my granny's apartment and I learned, object by object, that life isn't made more meaningful by 'things'. The more you have, the more junk you leave behind for others to sort out. I realised how generous it is to those we leave behind to live neatly and lightly.

Despite the reality that we can take nothing with us when we die, not even our bodies, we spend most of our lives holding onto things, people, places, our work and our histories as if they confirm our existence. Humans are walking velcro. The Buddhists call this 'attachment' and, far from it bringing us joy, it only heralds pain when we grasp the temporary nature of all things.

To live with less suffering, therefore, Buddhism encourages us to release our hold on things, and to practise detachment. The difference between attachment and non-attachment is the distinction between admiring a beautiful flower in nature and picking it. A friend of mine has a little girl who, when she sees a beautiful flower, kisses it. *This* is non-attachment.

Nonetheless, my sisters and I were attached to different objects that reminded us of Granny Bee. I wanted her hand-written green recipe book with her *schmaltz*y recipes. Her garlic press. Her egglifter. Her red glass salad bowl. My mother offered me her dining-room table and chairs around which I'd eaten hundreds of crispy meals.

It cost a fortune, but I had them shipped back to Australia. I hoped someday her table would be the centrepiece around which we'd build our own home.

After the euphoria of our homecoming wore off, like that instant rush of regret after you've succumbed to your ex's charm, you realise that you've been seduced by memory. It's not to be trusted. It is, after all, a hopeless romantic. It always tells half a tale. Memory had forgotten the high walls, the stress in suburban streets, the road rage, the blistering poverty and the homelessness which had made it hard to live there in the first place. Back home, my anxiety beanstalked overnight. I decided that though I'd missed much, I hadn't missed these things. It had been hard to leave all I'd loved so deeply, but I'd learned to live separately from them. Miserably at first, but I'd survived. I'd broken through.

With the understanding distance had given me, I could see that Australia is like the well-dressed, well-mannered kid who comes from a nice family, who won't embarrass you in public. Ask how it's feeling and you'll hear, 'It's all good, mate,' though you won't always get the truth. South Africa is like that crazy kid from the wrong side of the tracks you're always hoping is going to win the Nobel Prize or the Oscar. It's troubled and self-destructive and you pray someday it's just going to settle down with a nice girl. It wears its heart, poverty and lost generations on its sleeve. And just like I could never have married hyperactive Max or the Marxist activist because I didn't want to raise children in the chaos of madness or revolution, I had to concede that we, like the patient turtle, had chosen a spot of peaceful earth far from the frenzy of a highway or the precarious pathways of hungry wolves in which to bury our eggs.

After four weeks we left again, and the wrench was raw and fresh and bloody. I spent weeks recovering back in Sydney, wondering whether I was a South African who dreamed I was Australian or an Australian who dreamed I was South African.

RETURN

Like in the parable of Chuang Tzu, who dreamed he was a butterfly and, when he awoke, did not know if he was a man who had dreamed he was a butterfly or a butterfly who was dreaming he was a man, I made my home for a time in the overlaps.

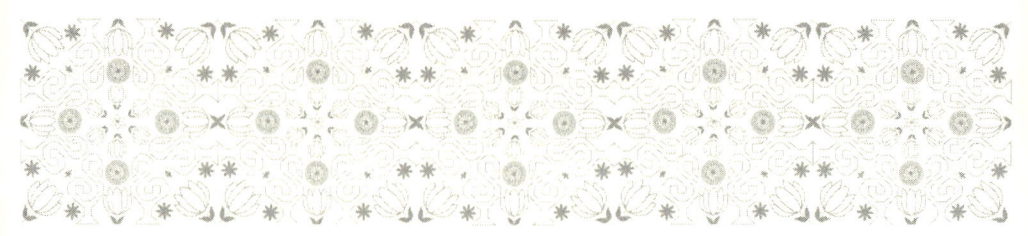

59
Roots

Lovers don't finally meet somewhere,
They're in each other all along.
RUMI

If I had a dollar for every time I've been asked why I decided to get married after eight years with Zed, two kids and an emigration, at roughly the same point in a relationship at which others are getting divorced, I'd never have to scramble for small change for a coffee again. I'd just call into the intercom to tell my personal barista to bring it up to the top deck.

Even when I explain how it happened my friends still give me a 'But I still don't get it... you were *never* getting married...' And it's true, I never was. Frankly, I'd never understood the appeal of a husband, which, much like certain venereal diseases, is very hard to get rid of once you've got it.

But sometime during our 'initiation' period in Australia, at round about the three-year mark, Zed and I had had (another) particularly unpleasant fight, around a major issue like whose turn it was to take out the garbage or clean the cat litter. I stormed east into our bedroom, fuming. He snarled off westwards muttering under his breath. It was a common scenario that had played out too many times since we'd immigrated.

But then, suddenly, he called me.

'What do you want?' I yelled.

'Just come here.'

'No, if you want to talk to me, you come here,' I screeched.

'Just come here,' he replied. 'Please.'

Something in the tone of how he called me nudged past my irritation and found its way to a gentleness I had so forgotten between us. I got up and followed his voice. He was standing outside pointing to the sky. Okay, I know this sounds totally clichéd and tacky – but there was a rainbow arched across the sky of the late afternoon. Except, take my word for it, this was no brown paper bag rainbow, it was the most totally glamorous air-brushed supersized Hollywood-special luminous eyebrow of light I'd ever seen. Like God was trying to make a point or something.

Whew. Fuck. Wow. We paused. Zed and I sank onto the back stairs of the rented house that we had both come to hate – because a) it wasn't ours and b) it was hard to love a place that always smelled of poo – and watched the rainbow, softened by its presence which seemed somehow connected to all things we'd lost and were yet to discover. Somewhere in the hush of early evening raspberry light and the reek of sewage, he put his hand in mine and said, 'It's going to be okay.'

I turned and faced this man who, just a short time ago, I could in a fit of ego-driven pique have walked out on and I looked into his kind face. I allowed myself to receive the comfort of those words: *It's going to be okay*. All the hardship of our three years in lonely exile stood back and made way for consolation. I felt a huge sob break from my throat and, when I put my arms around Zed, I reeled in the long and hard yards we had walked together, spooling in the times in which we'd forgotten to speak to each other with tenderness, and tuck away all our failures to be tolerant and gentle with one another.

Beneath that *schmaltzy* rainbow I saw that, despite how pathetic, desperate and horrible I had been over the past few years and how little I had come to love myself, Zed still loved me. And if he loved me at my worst, maybe he always would. He would never desert me or forsake me. He would be present and patient and would hold me in my suffering, just like God promised Jacob. Like a piece of flotsam, his love kept bobbing to the surface, a driftwood of residual respect and affection that the tides of change and trauma and displacement had failed to sink. And in that moment, we embraced all the hardship and awfulness to compost in the earth of our relationship so something new could spring forth. I finally understood what Sherill had meant about including the poo or missing the lesson.

Sometime soon after that I said, 'I love you enough to marry you.'

A few months later, barefoot under a huge Moreton Bay Fig tree in Centennial Park with roots as deep as time itself, surrounded by a handful of new friends, most of whom were also immigrants, we promised to help each other grow and become the best people we could be. We asked those present to be witnesses to our commitment, and to support us to love one another through the times that lay ahead. We also asked them to help us clean up the mess before they left and to put all their rubbish in the bins provided.

There we made a spot of earth a memorial, a tree our witness, and so began to claim a new history in our new land.

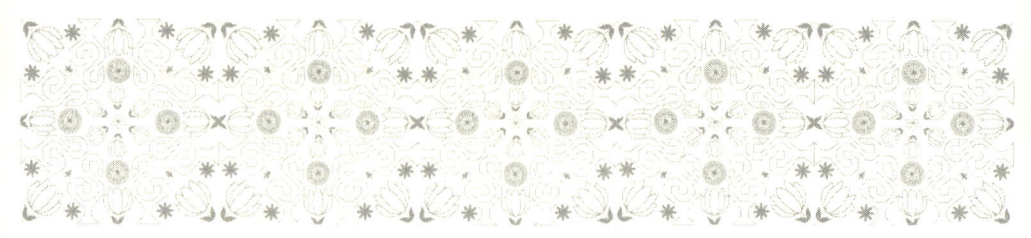

60
Sweet and sour

You can't expect both ends of the sugar cane to be as sweet.
CHINESE PROVERB

I have no detailed memories of the colossal bureaucratic mountain we had to scale to finally secure our Australian permanent residence. I vaguely recall numerous medical examinations, including an HIV test by a doctor who drew blood from my arm while having a conversation in Russian on a phone wedged between his ear and his shoulder. For weeks afterwards the streak of bruise down my forearm convinced me that men really shouldn't multi-task. When our permanent residence finally came through after a couple of years, we got Medicare and were eligible for free public schooling. These were two welcoming visas into the incredible generosity of Australian civic life and a great relief for a hypochondriac such as me.

For two more years, we waited out our time to apply for citizenship then navigated the bureaucratic maze to qualify, amassing a lengthy paper trail and developing a marathoner's stamina for filling in those little boxes in official documentation.

I've glossed over the many wonderful experiences of those years mostly because happiness tends to be so dull. But along the way, we met funny, soulful people who fed us prawns on the barbie, pavlovas and fairy bread, and who didn't make jokes about our accents. Each one helped us connect the dots of ourselves to a broader tapestry of Australian life. I felt like an Aboriginal painting that was finally coming into focus. Over time, the gaps contracted, and I began to feel more whole. Each connection weighed me down, held me to this sunburnt earth, taught me my place in the grand Aussie scheme of things. The kids swam between the flags, Jordan got stung by a bluebottle, I finally learned the words to 'Advance Australia fair', we got mauled by mozzies and tormented by February flies, we slipped, slopped and slapped, I learned how to play cricket, we bought a kayak, I purchased a sunhat with the Australian flag on it to wear on Australia Day. I began to dress right. People asked me for directions. I found ways of being helpful to others.

On 9 February 2006 we were invited to a citizenship ceremony at Randwick City Council where the mayor, Ted Seng, in his glorious Chinese accent, welcomed us as citizens of Australia.

I'd come unprepared with not a single tissue in my bag. I was deeply moved when the choir of young singers sang 'I still call Australia home'.

'Are you happy or sad?' Zed asked, offering me a crumpled Gloria Jean's serviette he'd found in a pocket.

'Both,' I said.

The relief I felt after the years of emotional and financial cost was a chocolate swirl in a gelato of sadness that bit my throat with the cold certainty that I was never 'going home', despite our dual citizenship and our twin passports. The way life had worked out, I wasn't going to be the one to arrive on my sisters' doorsteps with chicken soup. The hugs of my parents, sisters and friends would be annual, like dental check-ups. And the terrestrial sorrow of knowing that my parents would, in all likelihood, be laid to rest in earth only reachable in longing, sat indigestibly deep in my guts.

Over the years on our journeys back to South Africa, my homeland and I outgrew each other, like the trousers in my wardrobe that didn't quite fit anymore after a few months on my new eating plan. I resisted that knowledge, much like it pains me to toss out beloved items of clothing, because I didn't feel at home in Australia either. But after we'd returned a few times, I noticed that we'd begun a new history of *visiting* South Africa and *returning* to Australia.

As we touched down in Sydney after our fourth visit, I found myself saying, 'It's lovely to be home.'

'Oops, you said "home",' said Zed.

Did I?

I guess somewhere along the way I'd stopped struggling, and surrendered to the uncertainty. And maybe that's just the same as deciding to be happy.

'Well,' said Zed, waving his Australian flag and admiring our certificates of citizenship, 'it's certainly been a fucking expensive adventure.' And then we went to KFC to rejoice with Popcorn Chicken and Zinger Burgers.

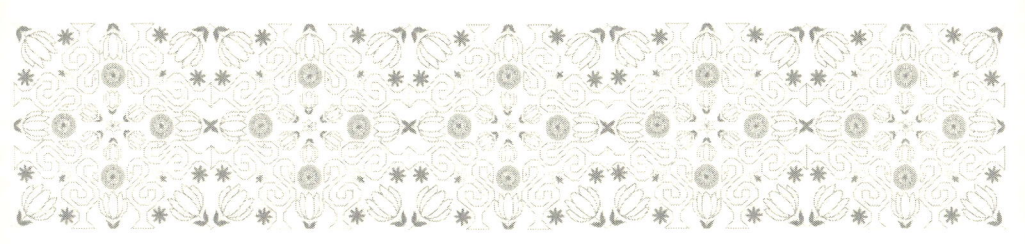

61
Coincidence #3

God often visits us but most of the time we are not at home.
FRENCH PROVERB

All things we care about must have a proper burial. That's why we take the time to lay people we love in the earth, or send them up in smoke instead of throwing them out with the garbage. We only get closure on what we mindfully surrender.

I didn't forget those women at WAGE. I thought I had – I'd banished them from conscious memory. But my body, it seems, was holding them in detention, amassing a library of testimonies without my knowledge or permission.

Where did I store these stories?

In my vagina.

You have to admit, that was a pretty good place to hide them – I mean, nobody thought to look there.

When you're struggling with continental changes and cultural upheavals, the last thing on your mind – take it from me – are cervical changes. The cervix is a shy piece of the female anatomy tucked away inside, doing us the favour of marking the difference between the womb and the vagina. Frankly, I wouldn't know my cervix from my pancreas having never actually *seen* it. The only way then to keep track of its changes is to make sure one marks those exciting annual visits to the GP on one's calendar for what is squeamishly called the Pap smear.

While most mothers can, at any given time, give a detailed description of every inch of their children's bodies, including the shape, colour and texture of their every meal and bowel movement, we're correspondingly inattentive to our own. As the stress of becoming Australian citizens was exacting a visible toll on me, it seems as if micro-mayhem was being wrought at a cellular level too. But I had, to be perfectly honest, forgotten all about my cervix.

Maybe I'm just lucky, but I like to think that a third coincidence came to my rescue once again in the form of a letter. Not a purposely concealed one, like my *zaide*'s, but one that found me, against all odds.

It happened one morning while I was putting Jordan's lunch box into his preschool locker. A mum I didn't know came up to me. 'Are you Joanne Fedler?' she asked.

'Yes,' I gushed. 'Do I know you?' (When you're still trying to fit in and be noticed, an acknowledgement from a stranger elicits disproportionate gratitude.)

No, but she knew a friend of mine, who had mentioned that my son was at the same kindergarten as her daughter. It so happened that she was now living in the very house in Bronte for which we'd been screwed into paying $50 more a week when we first arrived.

'It's a lovely house,' I confirmed. We had moved twice since then. I wondered how she knew we'd lived there.

COINCIDENCE #3

And this is how: a letter had arrived for me at the Bronte address and she'd recognised my name since her friend had mentioned our children's common kindergarten. She brought it in for me the next day.

I had hoped for something exciting – perhaps a letter from Ilze. Instead it was a computer-generated reminder from the pathology lab that it was time for me to go for my next Pap smear.

Like most women, I don't anticipate my Pap smears with any degree of enthusiasm. They are an inconvenience wrapped in an indignity and I do wish some eager medical researcher would come up with a better way of sampling the cells on the old cervix and just win a Nobel Prize or something for the effort.

Yet prompted by this reminder, I zapped into my GP for my smear, asked her about her kids and grabbed a pamphlet on vasectomies on the way out to leave on Zed's pillow. A week later she called back. Could I please come in to discuss my results? 'Discuss' and 'Pap smear' do not, as far as I can see, belong in the same sentence. Nonetheless, our discussion revealed that I had CIN III, caused by the human papilloma virus, which many of us carry without knowing it. HPV can remain dormant, but in some cases it can develop into cervical cancer and I was just one cell change off the Big C. I was sent to a specialist who wore a bow tie. He explained that he'd chop off a bit of my cervix and do biopsies into my uterus to see if there was any cancer.

Oh my God, I'm too young to die, I thought. Thirty-seven is practically still a teenager, give or take a decade. Then I remembered Princess Diana died when she was only thirty-six.

WHEN HUNGRY, EAT

My granny's mother Doris also died at thirty-six, so apparently it's not too young at all and what made me think I was so special that I should live into my doddering eighties?

My good old friend, fear, thought all its *Chanukahs* had come at once. It arrived in a limo, and moved in with all its baggage. Every time I looked at my children, I shrivelled into reckless misery. I told Zed to marry the babysitter if I died. The kids really liked her.

In the days leading up to my operation, I cried, spoke to God and sorted out my affairs. Fear kept me awake, howling like a hungry ghost. Eventually I had heard all its tales, retold over and over and over again, I'd been harangued and nagged and cajoled, I was completely spent ... and at some point I just stopped listening. Enough! Enough. In that small moratorium, in which fear took a breath and all was quiet, I was able to clear a little space, the way a beam of sunlight can find its way through the thickest of tree cover. And I crawled in there just to get some peace.

There I was, powerless and vulnerable, just a speck of humanity with a bloody virus that had corrupted my cervix and was threatening to take everything away from me, and after all the *schlep* and drama of getting to Australia. Would I live long enough to see Uluru? The Great Barrier Reef? The final episode of *The Biggest Loser*? Maybe I'd be okay, but maybe I wouldn't. It wasn't actually my call. Memories sidled in around me, familiar, pungent. I knew this powerlessness well. I'd been unable to fight the tides of life before, wishing I could change things, wishing I was driving. *My sister was stabbed to death with a pair of scissors. I was raped, my mother was raped, my daughter was raped. Rape is not the worst thing. I just want him to say sorry. Shot in maintenance court in full view of the magistrate.*

Every face, every name came back to me, one by one.

COINCIDENCE #3

I'd been carrying those stories all along.

I guess my vagina had taken it personally every time a woman told me she'd been raped. I'd always known in theory that everything we take in has a consequence; not only the food we eat, but the stories we hear and the things we see. It's why I never watch *CSI* or horror movies. It's why I left South Africa. We live within a matrix of fractals. Of course the human body metabolises emotions which mirror their micro-cousins at a cellular – perhaps even an atomic – level. Suddenly, instead of being angry at my body for turning on me like this, I realised what a compassionate sensitive creature it is, how receptive and gentle and empathetic it is to all human pain. My body wasn't turning on me, it was tuning me in.

I called my wise sister Laura. She's a big Louise Hay fan, and I wanted to know what she thought. 'Just forgive yourself,' she said.

'For what?' I asked.

'For whatever you blame yourself for.'

The night before my surgery I lay in the bath and I put my hands over my belly, in the region where I imagined my cervix to be, and I considered what it was that I could possibly be blaming myself for. Nothing seemed obvious or conscious. But of course, important things rarely are. They are hidden in the world, and we have to find them.

I waited a bit. And then some more. All those long, hard, sad years at WAGE eventually rose and lined up in front of me. I didn't want to look too closely at them. I realised that if I did, I'd see that I really hadn't been able to save anyone. I hadn't held back the tragedies like Superman. I understood how much of a personal failure this had felt to me. I thought of all the women and children who were still being raped and abused and how I'd once imagined I'd be able to stop these terrible things from happening. Leaving South Africa was a final concession that I had, in fact, given up.

My powerlessness and sadness came right up to the surface, all my wretched emotions, one by one, the prisoners of my psyche, starved and embittered from their years in solitary confinement. And I said aloud, 'I forgive myself for not being able to prevent women from being raped. I'm sorry I was never able to stop the hurt and the pain.' And, turning to my anger, I said, 'I'm setting you free now, please leave.' I closed my eyes and pictured the red, throbbing anger, that made my adrenalin gallop and my blood scream whenever I'd heard a woman or child had been raped, just ebb away.

My whole body juddered, as if burping or hiccupping a bad meal out. Then something freaky happened. I heard myself say: 'And I forgive the men who have raped and hurt women. I hope they know what they did was wrong. I hope they can find happiness, and feel self-worth and love so they never have to hurt another woman again.'

And my head said, *You can't say that!'*

Well, I just did, my body said.

As these words rushed unbidden from my mouth, my whole body shook. I wept great, wrenching sobs, and I like to imagine that each one of those stories left me in huge heaves and shudders and quakes and tremors, like a dog shaking itself free of water. And when I finally stopped shaking my entire body was so still in a way that felt quite new and holy.

When that stillness had filled me up, I was soft and pliant, alive and very, very free. And I knew I wasn't going to die.

COINCIDENCE #3

Not now and not because of this. I knew God just wanted me to let it all go, because really, it was enough.

The next day I underwent surgery with faith that, whatever the outcome, I would find a way to handle it – the way would be revealed even though I couldn't yet see it. There are worse things in life than a hysterectomy or chemotherapy. All I knew was that I wanted to live a long and healthy life and actually, I didn't want Zed to marry our babysitter. I wanted to grow old with him, and I'd do whatever it took to get there ... and if not, well I'd have to figure that one out too. But not today.

I'm still very grateful that those biopsy results came back clear.

Of course we have no control over what the future holds. But we always have control over what we choose to let go.

Not long afterwards I made my first appointment with the Food Fascist. Sometimes we mothers just need a little nudge in the fanny to remember to look after ourselves too.

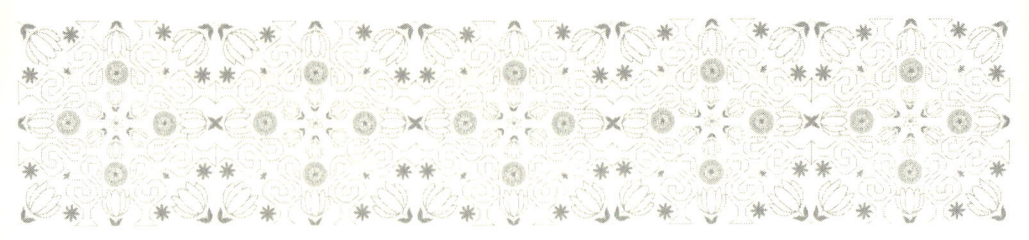

62
Angels

Every blade of grass has its angel that bends over it and whispers, 'Grow, grow.'
THE TALMUD

If our bodies are temples for our souls, I picture the vagina as its sweet little shrine. I like God's poetry, reminding me to do some internal housework and sweep my temple floors through a Pap smear scare. I'd been longing for a 'home', fixating on real estate, when what I needed was to bring God back into the architecture of my own skin, into the sanctuary of my bones. After babies, I knew my body was just a unit in God's timeshare scheme, but in my homesickness, I'd forgotten.

When the Jews wandered through the desert, they built portable residences or tabernacles known as *mishkan* in Hebrew, which has the same root as *Shekhina* or 'presence of God', reminding us that a home is a spiritual haven. In Jewish mystical thinking, *mishkan*, apart from being a place to hang your hat, also doubles up as a metaphor for the human soul. A home is just the physical structure into which we invite the holy

ANGELS

presence of God, and it doesn't matter whether that structure has skylights and lattices, or breasts and buttocks.

It took us five years of renting one place and then another to find an address for our *mishkan*. Zed's insomniac-driven internet searches late into the night brought him to an apartment a hundred metres from beautiful Coogee Beach. Soon he had his heart set on it. Since we couldn't afford it, I can only assume that the moon was in the seventh house and Venus aligned with Mars, causing a momentary dip in the property market to combine with the owner's desperation to sell. Whatever the case, before we knew it we were signing legal documents, though a thirty-year mortgage really makes it seem more like the bank's *mishkan* than ours. Ownership in any event is another fiction of the ego, as Aboriginal culture keeps trying to get us white fellas to understand. But, for the first time, we were free of landlords.

Zed led me into the apartment with its big old rooms and stained-glass windows and its sunroom with water views. In the lounge room, he said, 'Look up.' There on the old ceiling were four angels looking down on us.

Once we'd moved in, I unpacked boxes that hadn't been touched since our move from South Africa. I hammered dozens of nails into the walls and put up all my pictures. But our excitement was short-lived. As soon as night fell, a sobering reality settled, which perhaps shed some light on why we'd been able to afford this dream home. Above our bedroom was the upstairs unit's lounge room, which had a polished wooden floor. I know this because we got to enjoy every sound, from slippered footfall to gentle banter to raucous guffawing, to

Enja or Pink on the sound system, to *Prison Break* on TV as if we were in the same room. Nothing but a bit of sawdust seemed to separate us from the goings-on upstairs, some of which really didn't need an audience. To give you some idea of the insulation problem, the tenant upstairs overwatered his pot plant, which happened to be above my desk and my laptop died. Our *mishkan,* it seemed, was a dud.

We didn't sleep much. I wondered if we could turn the main bedroom into the dining room. I wondered if it would be odd if Zed and I camped in the lounge room for the rest of our lives. The owner of the upstairs unit, though obliged by law, refused to carpet the lounge room believing doing so would *spoil the aesthetic* of his investment property. I won't repeat the invective I flung in his direction at three am every morning except to say it went something along the lines of the Jewish curse, 'May you live in a house with a hundred rooms and may each room have its own bed, and may you wander every night from room to room and from bed to bed, unable to sleep'. Meanwhile, Zed quietly prepared the papers to take him to court.

Eventually, after months of disrupted sleep, as far from a sense of *mishkan* as I imagine a wife feels about the bedroom of her husband's infidelity, with our court hearing still months ahead of us, I contracted a sound specialist to install a false ceiling in our bedroom to insulate us from the noise above.

And that is how I met Wiremu Mutu. While this large twinkle of a man applied rubber matting and various other sound-absorbing materials, he told me stories about his Maori culture and traditions.

'You've got a lot of books,' he commented about my bookshelves. 'I don't read much,' he confessed, yet in our conversations he seemed familiar with all the spiritual theory I'd spent years reading.

ANGELS

I wondered whether it was hard for him to live away from New Zealand, and whether he missed home as much as I did. I hadn't always found Australians to be that friendly.

'My mother died when I was a boy and I never knew my father. I was moved around from relative to relative. So to me home is something you carry inside. I never feel far from home. Home is here,' he said, touching his chest.

My skin prickled. Sometimes God is so literal. This man had plainly been sent from above.

'I'll tell you a story,' he said. 'There was once a man in London headed for New York who asked a New Yorker what people are like in New York. The New Yorker asked, "Well, what are people like in London?" The man replied, "They're nasty and cold and unfriendly and no-one gives you the time of day." "Well, that's how people will be in New York," the New Yorker replied.'

And Wiremu Mutu carried on with his hammering as if he hadn't just told me kindly to stop being a whiney pain in the arse and get on with it. That I was, in fact, driving.

I started to laugh. I thought about my first three 'miserable' years in Australia when all I did was look back. How did I know whether or not people were friendly or unfriendly? I hadn't even been present in my own life. To paraphrase Goethe, I hadn't yet learned to trust myself, so I didn't know how to live.

Wiremu and I soon became close friends. His relationship with the earth and the wind and the sea made me look at things afresh. One day he asked if I wanted to learn to talk to the whales.

'How do I do it?'

'Ask them, "Are you here today?" And wait for them to answer.'

I tried, but I got no answers.

'You have to stop thinking. Your head keeps on getting in the way, doesn't it?' he laughed. 'Try asking with your heart.'

Sometime later he told me that after his mother died, he and siblings were dispersed amongst family members. All he had of his mother was a fork that had belonged to her which he always carried with him. But when he was twenty-three, he went out for a surf one day with the fork in his hand. It was misty, which, he explained, means the ancestors are close. He paddled out to where the sea was dark, and he threw that fork into the belly of the sea. 'I swam back to shore and for the first time, I was all alone inside myself,' he said. The burden of that steel, the only connection to his mother, was now the ocean's, and what he never had gently sank away.

'That day I walked on land as a free man,' he said.

There came a point on my new eating plan, and I can't identify exactly when it was, but certainly after I'd braved my hunger, changed my portion sizes and my habits, been tolerant with my failures, and picked myself up more than once and begun again. I'd come down a pant's size or two. I could feel my jaunty hip and sturdy collar bones. A twenty-year-old boy had winked at me mistaking me for a yummy mummy. Or maybe he just had something in his eye. And it dawned on me that I was never going back.

Never again would I be a person who orders fries with my hamburger. Never again would I eat a pie for lunch if there was sushi as an option. I'd never binge on chocolate and, if I did, I'd wake up the next morning and walk until my quadriceps told me to pick on another body part. If I ordered green curry, I'd eat only half, and keep the rest for tomorrow or for Zed. I found I preferred Chinese broccoli to rice, which I'd always eaten but never liked.

When I fronted up to the Food Fascist and was told I was 'obese', something irrevocable happened: I was offered a door into my own hunger. And when I stepped through, everything changed.

I began to see the metaphor I was inhabiting. I understood that learning to eat when I was hungry was just another way of making a home in a new place. Arriving in a strange country is both literal and figurative, physical and emotional. I'd begun in bewilderment, I'd wandered lost, I missed everything I'd left behind, always waiting to 'go home'. I'd had to cut out 'extras'. I'd learned that to live simply in units of moments was enough. Like Miriam, I started shrinking. I surrendered to the dissolution grief makes necessary. The hunger for the things I'd left behind eventually subsided. I celebrated a few precious luxuries and I enjoyed everything like I'd never enjoyed anything before. Like a beginner.

I'd counted the days, I'd paid my dues increment by increment. I realised that in all the time I'd been waiting for this state of limbo to be over, I'd made new friends, found new ways of being in the world, anchored new roots. I'd lost weight.

I understood that 'going back' was an illusion that prevented me from going forward. Inside my own body, I was already home.

The angels on my ceiling remind me to keep looking up and to stop looking back.

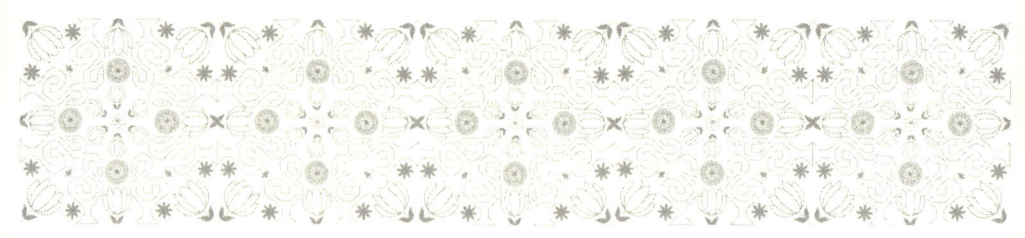

63
Swim

But don't be satisfied with stories, how things
Have gone with others. Unfold
Your own myth, without complicated explanation . . .
. . . Your legs will get heavy
And tired. Then comes a moment
Of feeling the wings you've grown,
Lifting.
RUMI

My swimming coach is a kind man with enormous shoulders. He is patient as I get into the water, which takes about five minutes punctuated with assorted involuntary squeaks and shrieks on my part. I've explained that I don't like cold water. He suggests that I shouldn't think too much because once you let the mind into the conversation, the body gets bullied.

'The mind has an aversion to the word "cold",' he says, 'when in fact, the body doesn't mind so much.'

It turns out he teaches theology to schoolgirls during the week and stroke correction to big girls like me on the weekends. Patience is most certainly his virtue as he shows me, time and time again, how to position my elbow, keep my fingers slightly apart and offers me the helpful suggestion that I should breathe not on every third stroke, but whenever I feel the need. I like his flexibility.

So why have I come here? Well, for one thing, since I've dropped a few kilos, I don't look so bad in a bathing costume. I'm still on one-pieces, which are forgiving as things that cover the nasty bits tend to be. But I also decided it was time to learn how to swim properly. It struck me a while ago that I'd been sending the kids to swimming lessons for years but had neglected to learn to swim properly myself. I needed some guidance on the mechanics of it all and, after a few short weeks under my coach's tutelage, the water has become a much friendlier place.

However, he told me the other day that he can only take a student so far.

'What do you mean?' I inquired. I certainly paid for a whole course and would like to be taken all the way, so to speak.

'It's one thing to show a person the correct posture and movement, but I cannot teach the most important thing, which is how your own body feels in the water. That's something each person has to find out on their own. It's a very personal relationship – how our arms, legs and torso feel moving through the water. No-one can tell you how to feel at home in the water.'

Don't you just love these overlaps?

Whether we're learning breaststroke, or healthier eating habits, or how to fit in, or the many ways there are to feel

God's gentle guidance, once we know the 'rules', we have to make it our own journey.

What others can teach us through their experiences is only useful to a certain point, and when we recognise where that point is, that's when our authentic experience begins. It becomes a fork in the road of our consciousness in which we turn and face inwards, and ask, 'How is it for you?'

To swim forward, we must knit links between the strangeness of what is before us in this moment and the ancient stories we carry inside us. These precious and delicate connections mend the leaks of our grief, helping us to speak of our history so we can see the colours of all the rivers that run in our veins. So that we can know what it means to talk of things that make us cry for reasons only the blood understands.

Kahlil Gibran says in *The Prophet*, 'Deep is your longing for the land of your memories'. The longing for what has passed is our deepest hunger, and we must feed it enough. If we overindulge it, we lose where we are in this moment. But if we starve it, our stories are lost.

Over the many years we've been in Australia, I'm still learning the steps in this strange dance between the past and present, here and there. Sometimes I manage them with grace, but I stumble often too.

It's not easy to be absent from important moments in your family's story. I've been far away while my father's been ill and had surgery to have a kidney removed. We've never been at any of my niece Jenna's eight birthday parties. Violet died suddenly when she was seventy, at a time in her life when she should have just been easing into her retirement, and guess who wasn't at the funeral? A few years later, Nthabiseng, whose nappies I used to change, lost her eight-year-old son in a car accident, and I had to call her over the phone, when all I wanted was to fold her in my arms. A well-loved professor of mine, Mike Larkin, was stabbed to death walking home one evening. I put a message up on Facebook. Friends have had babies, divorces and chemotherapy. I've missed crises and dramas and funerals. My parents are getting older. Across the ocean, I lie awake with sleepless dreams of family celebrations around the Shabbat table.

In Australia, my children wake up each day just as the sun goes down in Africa. They've grown up without grandparents, aunts or cousins. Our family gatherings are modest, often just the bones (me, Zed, the kids) with no extra *schmaltz* of extended family. But we've made special friends in Australia; the Kahns and others who've become our chosen 'family' and who share our joys and sorrows. We've learned how to rely on friends and how to ask for help. We call home, we email, we put pictures up on Facebook, we Skype. We try to keep the connections going, we feed the hunger of our loss, and we get by. You never feel full, but eventually it becomes 'enough'.

Home, I've come to understand, is as much a history as it is a geography. It's a place on the inside that holds us steady, that coiled thread of memories that anchors us to all that has passed. Home is where we light our Sabbath candles and dish up our chicken soup. Home is where we cry for the past we've left behind. Home is wherever we are now. And we can invite people to be our family, because love is enough to bring people together in loneliness.

When we physically depart the soil on which our feet first stood, and we leave behind the sunlight of our childhood, the jacaranda trees that marked our spring, we lose a million unseen things, especially the stories of how we came into being. They do not travel well, on the whole. They fray.

Ilze said the universe hates a vacuum and soon fills it.

Ilze was wrong. The universe contracted when I left South Africa and the places left by my parents, sisters and special friendships have never been filled. That hunger still lingers but I don't want to find substitutions. I've learned to be patient with that hunger. It is precious. Each time I return to South Africa I savour everyone like a taste of the most delicious *schmaltz*y treat, and I carry the sustenance back with me to Sydney, loving things even more for the smallness of what I've been given.

It's only taken me eight years in Australia and four years on a new eating plan to understand that being far away from those we love is just a symbol of how far away we are from the self that we can learn to love better.

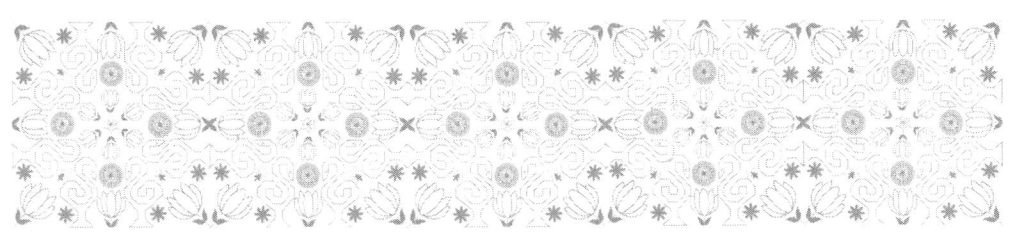

64
Digest

Eating is human, but digestion is divine.
IRANIAN PROVERB

Shannon asks if I know what cattle, goats, giraffes, yaks, water buffalo, deer, camels, alpacas, llamas, wildebeest and antelope all have in common.

'Ummm, they're all animals?' I offer.

She rolls her eyes. 'Duh ... but what else?'

I think for about three seconds and then give up.

'They all have four stomachs.'

I consider the immense value of a public school education in Australia and inform Shannon that this is indeed marvellous information.

'And do you know what these animals are called?' she asks.

I take what I consider to be a rather inspired stab. 'Four-stomached animals? Quadragasts?'

'Muuuum,' she tosses her head crossly. 'They're called ruminants.'

What a wonderful metaphor she's given me to end this story. Rumination, denoting the thorough digestion of yaks and cows, also means thoughtful pondering or meditating, which, like digestion, is a process through the gut of the soul, without beginning or end.

The cycle of digestion is a perfect micro-pattern of life. Just as the body absorbs food, so the mind and the heart assimilate all we take in. We have to let our experiences sink deep into our guts until we can absorb them into our bodies, our bones, our imagination, and our spirits. We need patience to draw out the nutrients, to find the meaning in each thing that is there to wake us up if we are present to meet it. And then we must let go of the hurt, the pain, the guilt, the shame, just as the body does, reminding us that it is a simple recipe: keep the good and let go of the bad, lest we become spiritually constipated.

Digestion needs time.

Time is nature's anaesthetic. Time is a measurement of healing. It's in no hurry and you can't rush it. It disengages grudges and unmoors us from the harbour of our grief. Time lets all our emotional prisoners out on parole. It allows the hurt to scab over, the rawness to subside. Time shifts us, rearranges the co-ordinates of our selves. And you, who once said 'I will never forget', find someday the untruth of that despair and say instead, 'I thought this day would never come'.

The day I first stood in front of the Food Fascist, I couldn't imagine that someday I'd find myself with a number pinned to my singlet in a crowd, ready to run a ten-kilometre race (all Zed's idea). I crossed the line almost last, me and the guy with the prosthetic, but I finished. Who could have predicted that exercise would become a secret love affair my body was having behind my back? That one day I'd just wake up and find my body had started to crave it, like it used to crave salt and vinegar chips.

When we left South Africa, my father made it clear that he'd never visit Australia: too far away and too long to sit on a plane, etcetera. Seven years later, he ate his words and made the trip, which apparently 'wasn't so bad after all'. He took in the simplicity of the beach on our doorstep, the quiet paradise of endless laundry and housework and healthy children bickering, the sunshine and the good humour of ordinary Australians having a barbie and a beer. It doesn't take much to get my dad to cry. He was proud of what we'd created after all we'd sacrificed and left behind. 'This is *nachas*. I'm glad I waited long enough to see you settled and happy in this place,' he declared, echoing his grandfather's words to his son, my *zaide*, that he would have forwarded the letter when he heard his son was happy and settled in his new home. I finally understood my father's reluctance to visit over all those years. Parents just can't bear to see their children suffer.

I never thought the day would come when I'd care about politics in Australia. But Zed and I were eligible to vote for the first time in the election in which Kevin Rudd took over from John Howard. The apology to the Aboriginal people made me proud to be a human being. We can all learn something from a gesture of forgiveness because the soul craves to care about something more than just itself.

I never thought someday I'd be making my living as an author. But being forced away from the harsh demands of WAGE, I finally buckled down and finished a book I'd been working on since Hedgebrook. And I found my place as a writer under the Australian sun.

To mark our seven years in Australia, I went on a bushwalk to meet this land with Uncle Max Dulumunmun, an Aboriginal elder. He explained that in Aboriginal culture, nothing is presumed. Before soil is taken from an anthill, ask permission by placing meat or honey on top. If the ants have abandoned it, you are welcome to use it. But always ask. For each thing has a spirit that is alive in this world, whether we can see it or not.

Some days later, I took the jar of shells we'd collected over our seven years in Australia and returned them to the ocean. We'd not thought to ask permission to take them. I don't know why we insist on picking things up and keeping them when we have no use for them, when they do not belong to us.

And seven and a half years after we arrived in Australia, we made a pilgrimage to Uluru, that sacred rock. We fretted about the tourists climbing it, especially when there's a sign at the base asking people not to out of respect for Aboriginal tradition. Zed reminded me of why we'd come. To pay *our* respects. So we marked the earth with our footprints around its base; we stood under its shadows and we watched its colours change.

Then we each in turn thanked God for guiding us to this place and asked the great and ancient spirits of this land for permission to be here.

Finally, I never thought the day would come when I'd think of the Food Fascist with anything resembling fondness. But sixteen kilos lighter, I now recognise the immense kindness and compassion it takes not to feed people's bullshit and capacity for self-deception. It's not easy to make people pay attention to the small broken promises they're accumulating every time they reach for something to eat.

Though I can't believe I'm thinking this, she's not so different from Ilze. Both of them refuse to tell anything but the truth. She gave me the kick up the arse I needed to stop pretending it was okay to be unmindful when carefulness, reflection and moderation are great and important human values, not just sensible habits to apply when eating. She taught me to slow down, to take every experience one bite at a time, moment by moment. I learned to pause and in those pauses to understand that I'm free to choose what to do next. I've learned to gently disentangle myself from my fear, my guilt and my nostalgia, like a mother might finally push her toddler from her in a gesture of loving empowerment.

Losing weight and emigrating helped me to recognise hunger in all its forms, not only in myself but in others. I see hunger wherever I turn. Hunger for love. Hunger for understanding. Hunger for grandchildren. Hunger for justice. Hunger for recognition. Hunger for kindness. Hunger for intimacy. Hunger for safety. Hunger for tolerance. Hunger for peace. We have a hungry, hungry world.

We have to learn how to nourish this hungry world.

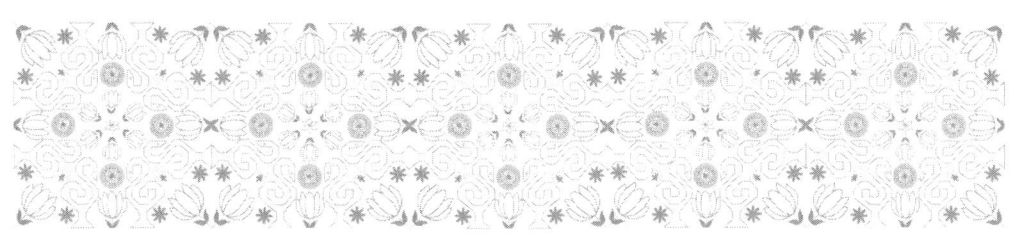

Epilogue

The more you know, the less you need.
ABORIGINAL SAYING

At Dolphin Point, at the end of my street, stands a memorial of three interlocking heads bowed in grief, exposed to the scatty sea winds and stinging rains, in memory of the eighty-three Australians who died in the terrorist attack in Bali on 12 October 2002. This spot, where the satiny bolt of ocean rolls out to the spine of the horizon, is a good place to come and stand when I'm homesick and doubt-ridden. Here I can hold the mustard seed of my problems up against the wide sky encompassing the million tragedies, losses and mysteries of human life and let them go, little dandelion tufts of suffering into the wild wind. When I come to this open place, I am able to cup everything I have lost softly in the palm of my hand, braver and stronger for knowing that I survived losing them. It's just another one of those sweet coincidences that *oz* in Hebrew means strength.

This monument is a daily reminder that safety is an illusion. It's not a fixed place, nor a destination. Safety isn't somewhere 'out there', it's 'in here'. It's what we touch when we feel: *anochi imach*. I am with you. There is nowhere 'safe' on this fragile, temporary earth. The only safety we can trust is the shelter within ourselves where we tend the sacred, delicate flame of faith.

The toughest spiritual challenge we each face is how to hold onto faith, especially when bad things happen – as they invariably will. Viktor Frankl calls this capacity we have for spiritual renewal in the face of fear 'tragic optimism'. People we love may be diagnosed with horrible illnesses, die in car accidents or become paralysed or rendered incapacitated. These things may indeed happen to us. Life is uncertain. All we can know is that the uncertainty remains, flickering like an infinite ember in the kiln of this incarnation.

Faith steers us towards finding a shelter amidst the uncertainties of life. It guides us to a momentary foothold – and it's just that, momentary, before something knocks us off balance and we must scramble to locate it once again. Like trawling for an elusive nugget under water, seeing it, losing it, seeing it again, faith is the labour of returning to this search. This nurturing of the space hallowed by our attention is a daily affair. A moment-by-moment devotion.

We do it one breath, one mouthful at a time.

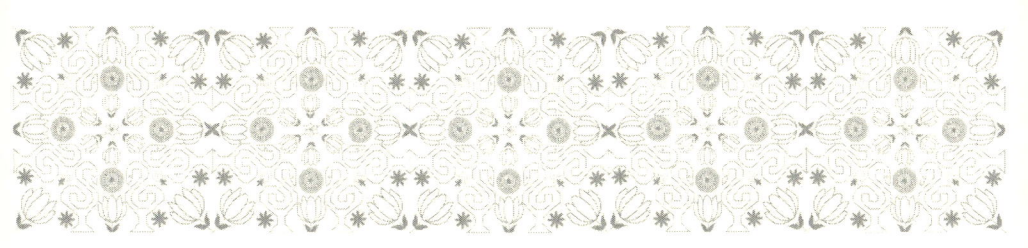

Appendix

An eating meditation, or spiritual principles, for losing weight, leaving home or letting go

> *Traveller, there are no paths.*
> *Paths are made by walking.*
> ABORIGINAL SAYING

I like principles. They retune the mind in the way we might reset a watch that has been set for another time and place. They are places to come back to. As we each follow our path of choice, whether it be *The Way*, the *Halacha* of the Torah, the *Qur'an*, the Noble Eightfold Path, or a twelve-step program, the *Kabbalah* tells us that there is also a personal path, called *Nativ*, which must be forged by each of us personally, day by day, in each moment we make sacred by our awareness.

Here are some of the principles I've learned in the course of my journey, reminding me that how I do anything is how I do everything:

1. *When hungry, eat:* Let your needs guide you.
2. *Always ask:* Make no assumptions. Come with a Beginner's Mind. Be open to what is strange and uncertain.
3. *Make healthy choices:* There are consequences to what and how we choose.
4. *Thank the food:* Everything we have is the result of sacrifices others have made. We can practise gratitude for whatever is in front of us.
5. *There is always enough:* Have faith that everything you need in this moment has been given. Trust that there will be more when you need it.
6. *Savour the taste:* Taste, like the breath, happens in the present moment. Celebrate every mouthful with the question: How is it for me?
7. *Slow down:* The spaces between mouthfuls, the hunger between meals, grows our awareness of our true nature.
8. *Digest:* The body knows what to do. Trust it. Give it time.
9. *Flush and Wash:* Let go of what you don't need to hold onto anymore.
10. *Begin again:* Come back, return, recommit.

APPENDIX

A Recipe for chicken soup (low *schmaltz*)

three large onions, sliced
one leek, sliced
one teaspoon of olive oil
four sticks of celery, chopped
one large chicken
a litre of water
one zucchini, sliced
three carrots, sliced
a few florets of cauliflower

a piece of pumpkin, diced
one turnip, sliced
one tomato, quartered
a sprinkle of turmeric
one cup of chicken stock
  (or one to two stock cubes
  in same amount of water)
ten peppercorns
three bay leaves

1. Find someone in need of chicken soup.
2. Brown the onions and leek in a teaspoon of olive oil.
3. Add the chopped celery. Thank it for its low kilojoule count.
4. Add the chicken and turn it occasionally to brown the skin. Thank the chicken for its sacrifice.
5. Add the water. Have a glass or two to drink while you're at it to make up your eight glasses of daily intake.
6. Add the zucchini, carrots, cauliflower, pumpkin, turnip, tomato and turmeric and let it all come to the boil. Add the chicken stock (or cubes in water), the peppercorns and bay leaves. Praise them for their co-operation in bringing it all together.
7. Step away from the pot and let the ingredients do their work for half an hour. Don't *kibbitz* the soup.
8. Switch off the pot and let it cool down before putting it in the fridge. Don't rush the soup. All things need time to cool off.
9. Later all the *schmaltz* will have formed a layer on the top. Scrape off and throw away.
10. Reheat the soup. Bless it and all who eat it.

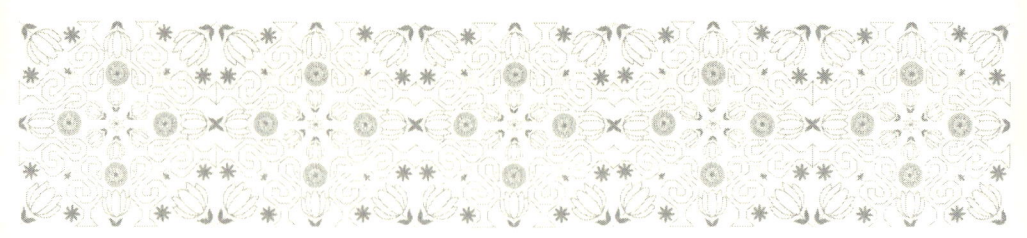

Stuff I read while I was hungry

Allende, Isabel, *Aphrodite: The love of food and the food of love,* Flamingo, 1998
Arenson, Gloria, *Five Simple Steps to Emotional Healing,* Fireside, 2001
Baldwin, Christina, *The Seven Whispers: Listening to the voice of spirit,* New World Library, 2002
Batchelor, Stephen, *Buddhism Without Beliefs: A contemporary guide to awakening,* Bloomsbury, 1997
Bays, Brandon, *The Journey,* Thorsons, 1999
Bennett, Merit, *Law and The Heart: A practical guide for successful lawyer/client relationships,* The Message Company, 1997
Berg, Leila, *The God Stories: A celebration of legends,* Francis Lincoln Limited, 1999
Binder, David, Paul Bergman and Susan Price, *Lawyers as Counselors: A client-centred approach,* West Publishing, 1991
Boorstein, Sylvia, *That's Funny, You Don't Look Buddhist: On being a faithful Jew and a passionate Buddhist,* Harper, 1997
Boss, Pauline, *Ambiguous Loss: Learning to live with unresolved grief,* Harvard University Press, 2000
Bria, Gina, *The Art of Family: Rituals, imagination and everyday spirituality,* Dell Publishing, 1998
Bryson, Bill, *Down Under,* Doubleday, 2000
Cameron, Julia, *The Artists' Way,* Pan Books, 1995

Campbell, Joseph with Bill Moyers, *The Power of Myth*, Anchor Books, 1991
Chah, Ajahn, *Living Dhamma*, The Sangha, Bung Wai Forest Monastry, 1992
Chatwin, Bruce, *The Songlines*, Vintage, 1998
Chopra, Deepak, *The Seven Spiritual Laws of Success*, Bantam Press, 1996
Chopra, Deepak, *How to Know God: The soul's journey into the mystery of mysteries*, Rider, 2000
Choquette, Sonia, *Soul Lessons and Soul Purpose*, Hay House, 2007
Claxton, Guy, *The Heart of Buddhism: Practical wisdom for an agitated world*, Thorsons, 1990
Dalai Lama, His Holiness, *Ancient Wisdom, Modern World: Ethics for a new millenium*, Little, Brown & Company, 1999
Dalai Lama, His Holiness, *An Open Heart: Practicing compassion in everyday life*, Hodder, 2001
Dawkins, Richard, *The God Delusion*, Bantam Press, 2006
Dowrick, Stephanie, *Forgiveness and Other Acts of Love*, Penguin Books, 1997
Dowrick, Stephanie, *Choosing Happiness: Life and soul essentials*, Allen & Unwin, 2005
Dreher, Diane, *Women's Tao Wisdom: Ten ways to personal power and peace*, Thorsons, 1998
Ensler, Eve, *The Vagina Monologues*, Villard, 1998
Epstein, Mark, *Going to Pieces Without Falling Apart: A Buddhist perspective on wholeness*, Thorsons, 1998
Estes, Clarissa Pinkola, *Women Who Run with the Wolves*, Ballantine Books, 1992
Fedler, Chaya, 'Falling Leaves', translated from Yiddish by Rachel Rose Abramowitz (my aunty Rae)
Fedler, Joanne and Ilze Olckers, *Ideological Virgins and Other Myths: Six principles for legal revisioning*, Justice College and the Law, Race and Gender Research Unit, 2000
Fedler, Solomon, *Shalechet*, S. Fedler & Co., 1969
Fields, Rick with Peggy Taylor, Rex Weyler and Rick Ingrasci, *Chop Wood, Carry Water: A guide to finding spiritual fulfilment in everyday life*, Penguin, 1984
Fordham, Frieda, *An Introduction to Jung's Psychology*, Penguin, 1953

Frankiel, Tamar, *The Gift of the Kabbalah: Discovering the secrets of heaven, renewing your life on earth*, Jewish Lights Publishing, 2001
Frankl, Viktor, *Man's Search for Meaning*, Pocketbooks, 1946
Free, Pamela J., *Come Home to Your Body*, Llewellyn Publications, 1997
Friedman, Lenore and Susan Moon (eds), *Being Bodies: Buddhist women on the paradox of embodiment*, Shambhala Publications Inc., 1997
Gibran, Kahlil, *The Prophet*, Heinemann, 1926
Gilbert, Elizabeth, *Eat, Pray, Love*, Bloomsbury, 2006
God (presumably), The Old Testament
Gold, Rabbi Shefa, *Torah Journeys: The inner path to the promised land*, Ben Yehuda Press, 2006
Granny Bee's handwritten recipe book
Greenwood, Dr Michael and Dr Peter Nunn, *The Paradox of Healing: Transforming your relationship with illness*, Prion, 1996
Guiliano, Mireille, *French Women Don't Get Fat: The secret of eating for pleasure*, Chatto & Windus, 2005
Hahn, Thich Nhat, *Being Peace*, Rider, 1987
Hay, Louise, *You Can Heal Your Life*, Hay House, 1984
Hay, Louise, *Reflections on Your Journey*, Hay House, 1995
Horne, Donald, *The Lucky Country*, Penguin Books, 1964
Horwitz, Nola, *The Full Circle: From Australia to South Africa and back*, Jewish Museum Community Services, 2006
Huntley, Rebecca, *Eating Between the Lines: Food and equality in Australia*, Black Inc., 2008
Jenkins, Peggy J., *Nurturing Spirituality in Children*, Beyond Words Publishing, 1995
Jonsson, Gudrun, *Gut Reaction*, Vermilion, 1998
Kennedy, Helena, *Eve Was Framed: Women and British justice*, Vintage, 1992
Khema, Aya, *Being Nobody, Going Nowhere: Meditations on the Buddhist path*, Wisdom Publications, 1987
Kingsolver, Barbara, *Animal, Vegetable, Miracle: Our year of seasonal eating*, Faber & Faber, 2007
Kinsey, Alfred C, *Sexual Behaviour in the Human Male*, WB Saunders Company, 1948
Kornfield, Jack, *A Path with Heart: A guide through the perils and promises of spiritual life*, Rider, 1994

Kornfield, Jack, *After the Ecstasy, the Laundry: How the heart grows wise on the spiritual path*, Rider, 2000
Krishnamurti, J, *On Fear*, Harper San Francisco, 1995
Krog, Antjie, *Country of My Skull*, Random House, 2002
Kubler-Ross, Elisabeth, *On Death and Dying*, Tavistock Publications, 1970
Larkin, Geri, *Stumbling Toward Enlightenment*, Celestial Arts, 1997
Leunig, Michael, *A Common Prayer: A cartoonist talks to God*, HarperCollinsReligious, 1990
Leunig, Michael, *Poems, 1972–2002*, Viking, 2003
Leunig, Michael, *The Lot in Words*, Viking, 2008
Maltz, Maxwell, *Psycho-Cybernetics*, Prentice-Hall, 1960
Mogel, Wendy, *The Blessing of a Skinned Knee: Using Jewish teaching to raise self-reliant children*, Penguin Books, 2001
Moore, Thomas, *Care of the Soul: How to add depth and meaning to your everyday life*, Piatkus, 1992
Myss, Caroline and Norman Shealy, *The Creation of Health*, Three Rivers Press, 1988
Myss, Caroline, *Anatomy of the Spirit: The seven stages of power and healing*, Bantam Books, 1997
Myss, Caroline, *Why People Don't Heal and How They Can: A practical programme for healing body, mind and spirit*, Bantam Books, 1998
Myss, Caroline, *Sacred Contracts: Awakening your divine potential*, Bantam Books, 2001
Myss, Caroline, *Invisible Acts of Power: Personal choices that create miracles*, Free Press, 2004
Myss, Caroline, *Entering the Castle: An inner path to God and your soul*, Free Press, 2007
Nairn, Rob, *Tranquil Mind: An introduction to Buddhism and meditation*, Carrefour & Dragon, 1993
Napthali, Sarah, *Buddhism for Mothers*, Allen & Unwin, 2003.
Northrup, Dr Christiane, *Women's Bodies, Women's Wisdom: The complete guide to women's health and wellbeing*, Piatkus, 1995
Peretz, Isaac Leib and Ruth R Wisse, *The IL Peretz Reader*, Yale University Press, 2002
Pogrebin, Letty Cottin, *Deborah, Golda and Me: Being female and Jewish in America*, Anchor Books, 1991
Rich, Adrienne, *The Fact of A Doorframe: Poems selected and new, 1950–1984*, Norton & Co., 1984
Rilke, Rainer Maria, *Letters to a Young Poet*, New World Library, 2000

Robbins, Anthony, *Awaken the Giant Within*, Simon & Schuster, 1992
Ruiz, Don Miguel, *The Four Agreements: A practical guide to personal freedom*, Amber Allen Publishing, 1997
Rumi, *The Essential Rumi*, Penguin Books, 1995
Schatz, Halé Sofia, *If the Buddha Came to Dinner*, Hyperion, 2004
Schultz, Mona Lisa, *Awakening Intuition: Using your mind–body network for insight and healing*, Bantam Books, 1999
Siegel, Bernie, *Living, Loving and Healing*, The Aquarian Press, 1993
Sparks, Allister, *The Mind of South Africa: The story of the rise and fall of apartheid*, Mandarin, 1990
Spieler, Marlena, *Jewish Cooking*, Hermes House, 2004
Suttner, Immanuel (ed.), *Cutting Through the Mountain: Interviews with South African Jewish activists*, Penguin, 1997
Tagore, Rabindranath, *Fruit-Gathering*, Macmillan, 1916
Toller, Eckhart, *The Power of Now*, Hodder, 2004
van der Post, Laurens, *A Mantis Carol*, Island Press, 1983
Walsh, Neale Donald, *Applications for Living from Conversations With God*, Hodder & Stoughton, 1999
Watts, Alan, *The Way of Zen*, Penguin Books, 1937
Williams, Patricia J, *The Alchemy of Race and Rights*, Harvard University Press, 1991
Wilson, Eric G, *Against Happiness*, Sarah Crichton Books, NY, 2008
Woolf, Virginia, *Moments of Being: Unpublished autobiographical writings*, Harcourt, Brace, Jovanovich, 1976
Zalman, Rabbi Shneur of Liadi, *The Tanya*, Kehot Publication Society, 1984

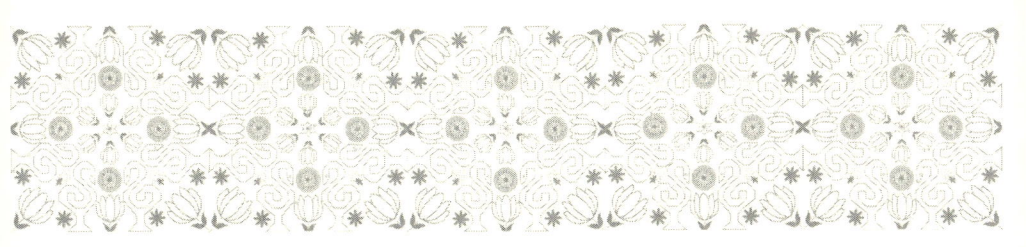

Glossary

AFL   Australian acronym for Australian Football League also referred to as 'Footy', especially popular in Victoria and South Australia

Amasi   Zulu or Xhosa for fermented milk that tastes like yogurt or buttermilk used in cooking

Anochi Imach   Hebrew, taken from the Old Testament (Genesis 28:10 – 32:3), literally meaning, 'I am with you'

Anzac Day   public holiday in Australia celebrated on 25 April in memory of the first major military action fought by Australian and New Zealand forces during the First World War (ANZAC stands for Australian and New Zealand Army Corps)

Barbie   Australian colloquialism, contraction of 'barbeque', generally an open-coal fire or gas flame to cook meat

Barmitzvah   coming-of-age ceremony celebrated by Jewish boys when they turn thirteen and are considered responsible adults

WHEN HUNGRY, EAT

Biltong spiced and cured dried raw meat eaten by South Africans. The word *biltong* is from the Dutch *bil* (rump) and *tong* (strip or tongue)
Blintze traditional Jewish food, a crepe that is either stuffed with cream cheese (sweet) or mince (savoury)
Bludger Australian slang for a lazy person
Bobba Yiddish for 'grandmother'
Boerewors South African sausage, literally 'farmers' sausage'
Bogan Australian slang for a person of low quality, unsophisticated or lacking class (analogous to US term 'redneck')
Boogy-board surfboard for catching waves
Braai South African term for a barbeque
Challah plaited sweet bread Jews eat on Sabbath
Channukah Jewish festival of Lights celebrated over eight days
Chassid(ic) a sect of Orthodox Jews that follows the Mosaic law strictly
Chuppah canopy traditionally used in Jewish weddings supported by four poles, symbolising the home the married couple will create – literally meaning 'canopy' or 'cover'
Chutzpah untranslatable Yiddish word for a mixture of charisma, cheek, audacity, shamelessness or gumption; not generally used in a pejorative way
'Die Stem' the official South African national anthem from 1957–94, literally 'The Call of South Africa'. Its words now form part of a hybrid national anthem together with '*Nkosi Sikelel' iAfrika*'
DOCS Australian acronym for Department of Child Services

360

GLOSSARY

EFTPOS Australian acronym for 'electronic funds transfer at point of sale', where a bank card can be used instead of a credit card or paying cash

Eina African expression for 'Ow' or 'Ouch'

Ein sof infinite, literally 'without end', a term used in the *Kabblah* to describe God's omnipresence

Fairy bread Australian traditional food eaten at children's parties where white bread spread with butter is then sprinkled with hundreds and thousands

Faribel Yiddish for grudge or resentment

Flat white Australian term for a coffee that is neither a latte nor a cappuccino

Floaties Australian term for 'water wings' or 'armbands' used by small children in the water so they don't drown

FlyBuys Australian customer loyalty reward system used by a chain of stores

Gefilte fish traditional Jewish fish balls made from minced deboned fish, popular in the Ashkenazi Jewish community; literally stuffed fish

Grundnorm German expression for core value of a civil legal system

Hadidah A type of large loud South African bird that looks like an Ibis

Halacha denotes the collective body of Jewish religious law, including biblical law, customs and traditions; often translated as 'Jewish Law', though more literally 'the path' or 'the way of walking', derived from the Hebrew word 'to walk'

'Hatikvah' national anthem of Israel, literally 'The Hope', written by Naphtali Herz Imber

361

Highveld	high plateau inland region of South Africa; geographical area comprising mainly northern South African provinces, opposite of the Lowveld because of elevation above sea level
Hoe gaan dit?	Afrikaans meaning 'How's it going?'
Kabbalah	Jewish mystical canon
Kashrut	Jewish dietary laws
Kibbitz	from Yiddish; to give unwanted advice or criticism or make unhelpful or idle comments especially to someone playing a game
Kneidel(ach)	Jewish dumplings made from matzo meal and schmaltz generally found in chicken soup
Latke	deep-fried potato pancake traditionally eaten by Jews on *Channukah*
Lekka	Afrikaans for 'good' or 'nice'
Lokshen	Yiddish for 'noodles'
Long Bay	a maximum security prison in Sydney
Lubavitch	branch of Chassidic Judaism with a leader or 'rebbe' based in Crown Heights in New York
Matza/o	unleavened bread Jews eat on Passover, in memory of the rapid exodus from Egypt where there was no time to wait for the bread to rise
Medicare	Government-sponsored public health service for Australian residents and citizens
Mensch	Yiddish for a humane, decent or good person
Mielie(s)	South African term for 'corn on the cob'
Mishkan	Hebrew, literally meaning 'residence' or 'dwelling place', denoting the portable 'tabernacle' or 'sanctuary' in which Jews worshipped God during their meanderings through the desert; also

GLOSSARY

	refers to any place or home in which one makes God's presence felt
Mohel	rabbi who performs Jewish ritual circumcision
Mozzies	Australian contraction of 'mosquitoes'
Nachas	an untranslatable Yiddish word for the pleasure Jewish parents derive from their children's success or invariable genius, good looks, brilliance, etc.
Nativ	Hebrew, literally meaning 'path', used in the Kabbalah to describe the individual path each person must forge in this life
'Nkosi Sikelel' iAfrika'	national anthem of South Africa, composed in 1897 by Enoch Sontonga, a Methodist school teacher; originally sung as a church hymn but later became a freedom song in political defiance of the apartheid government
Onkel	how you might pronounce 'uncle' with a Yiddish accent
'Op ons'	Afrikaans, literally 'on us' or 'cheers'
Ousie	Afrikaans for 'older sister'; colloquially used in referring to an older African woman; intended as a respectful name for an elder
Oz	Hebrew, literally meaning 'strength'
Pap	a traditional porridge made from ground maize and a staple food of the Bantu people of South Africa, often eaten together with meat
Pripetshok	Yiddish for 'hearth' or 'fireplace'
Rachmanut	Hebrew, literally meaning 'mercy' 'pity' or 'compassion'
Rachmonis	Yiddish word for someone in need of mercy, pity or compassion reserved for the pathetic and helpless
Rosh Hashana	Jewish New Year

363

Sangoma	African witchdoctor
Schmaltz	fat or fatty
Schmaltzy	fatty or colloquially used to describe an indulgence of sentiment as in a '*schmaltzy* movie'
Sefirot	Hebrew, plural of '*sefirah*', meaning 'enumerations'. *Kabbalistic* term referring to the ten attributes or emanations through which God reveals himself, comprising crown, wisdom, understanding, kindness, strength, beauty, victory, glory, foundation and kingdom
Shabbat	Jewish Sabbath celebrated from sundown on Friday night until the first three stars appear on Saturday night
Shebeen	illegal pub in townships in South Africa
Shekhina	Hebrew for the divine feminine presence of God, literally 'dwelling' or 'settling'
Shochet	Jewish ritual slaughterer who must slaughter animals for them to be considered 'kosher' by Jewish dietary law
Shevirat hakelim	*Kabbalistic* term literally meaning 'the shattering of the vessels', describing the moment when God's energy was dispersed through the universe
Shlep	Yiddish, to carry clumsily or with difficulty; an arduous journey
Slip, slop and slap	Australian campaign to prevent skin cancer by encouraging children to 'slip' on a t-shirt, 'slop' on sunblock and 'slap' on a hat
Snoek	fish common to South African waters
Shosholoza	hymn or chant-like song, sung traditionally by black labourers in South Africa, now also sung at sporting events
Shtetl	Yiddish for village
Shul	synagogue, Jewish place of worship

GLOSSARY

Superfund	Australian retirement investment
Tatts	Australian colloquialism, contraction of 'tattoos'
The Tanya	a compilation of *Chassidic* mysticism (*Kabbalistic* psychology and theology) compiled by Rabbi Schneur Zalman of Liadi and first published in 1797
Tay Sachs disease	or TSD is a genetic disorder that causes a progressive deterioration of mental and physical abilities in children from the age of six months and usually resulting in death around the age of four. There is currently no cure for the disease and there is a noticeable prevalence of the gene in Ashkenazi Jews from Eastern Europe
Tikkun Olam	*Kabbalistic* term for 'healing the world'
Toyi-Toyi	a Southern African dance, originally from Zimbabwe, that became famous for its use in political protests during the apartheid struggle
True blue	genuine Aussie, true to the flag
Tuchus	Yiddish for bum, bottom, butt
Tzimtzum	*Kabbalistic* term meaning 'contraction'
Uluru	Ayers Rock, sacred Aboriginal site in the Northern Territory of Australia
Villawood	Suburb of western Sydney, location of refugee detention centre
Voetsek	Afrikaans term for 'Get lost!'
Yarmulka	Jewish religious head-covering for men
Yizkor	Jewish memorial prayer for dead relatives said on the Day of Atonement (Yom Kippur)
Yom Kippur	Jewish Day of Atonement, fast from sundown to sunset
Zaide	Yiddish for 'grandfather'

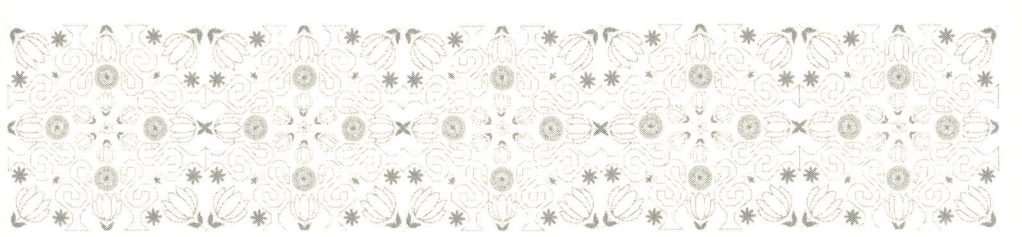

Acknowledgements

Two years after we left South Africa and after a long discussion about the heartache of leaving, my friend Denis Becket suggested I write a book about our experience of immigration.

'Too hard,' I'd responded.

I have no sensible explanation for why I didn't listen to myself. I mean, some things get better and easier with repetition. Sex, for example. Writing a book doesn't seem to. And this book – like a breach baby – hurt like hell coming out. I cried a lot. I had creative slumps. I was probably not very nice to be around quite a bit of the time.

Nonetheless, now that it's done, I am grateful to Denis for planting the seed. What began as a book about the losses of my heart, helped me to navigate the losses on the scale. And I'm not such a giddy fright in running shorts these days.

My parents have showered us with their love and support over the years, which has truly sustained us. I cannot imagine the generosity it took to surrender us and their grandchildren to the Antipodes. Thank you for every visit, phone call and email and for always holding us in spirit. Mom, Dad, Carolyn,

Laura, Dave and Jer, missing you never gets easier. Jenna – being so far away from you is 'suckish'.

I am thankful to all my teachers, past and present who came into my life in the guise of friends, nasty landlords, parents, children, clients at POWA, in-laws, illness, a pernickety dietician, tradesmen, Buddhists, rabbis, atheists, *Kabbalists*, cats and a flabby belly.

Without my *zaide*'s wonderful autobiography, *Shalechet*, and my Aunty Nola's book, *The Full Circle*, I'd have been bereft of so many stories from my family's history. And without my Aunty Rae's translation of my *bobba* Chaya's poems from Yiddish to English, I'd never have known my *bobba*'s heart. To all those people out there who want to write their life stories but don't think anyone will care, believe me, they will. Maybe only after you're long gone, but *they will care*. Write your stories.

My folks, sisters, Ilze, Thanissara and Zed read early drafts and their feedback and suggestions shaped and refined this book. Thank you for your time and input.

Hugs to Jo Paul for all her energy in getting this book to first draft. I am indebted to the wonderful Louise Thurtell for adopting me mid-way, her brilliant editorial suggestions and fighting for my title. Thanks to the editorial team at Allen & Unwin, in particular Joanne Holliman and Simone Ford, and to Ellie Exarchos for her beautiful cover design.

I am deeply thankful for families – genetic and chosen. In Australia, we are grateful for special friendships with the Segel-Friedmans (we'd be lost without you guys), Michelle and Phil, Kaaren and family, the Riesels, Lisa, Chad and Kaity, Emma, the Laxs, the Weiner-Angelopulos, Al and Lil Blank, the Altmans, Miri and Elozer and everyone else I have omitted to mention, but not on purpose. Please submit all your *faribels* to Allen & Unwin.

ACKNOWLEDGEMENTS

Jesse and Aidan – you are the tears in my smile, the rain in my desert, the vowels in my alphabet soup. You are the reason it all matters.

Zed, you are the fan on my hot day, the flyscreen on my window, the blessing in my disguise. Thanks for loving me when I was technically obese and for holding my hand through this journey. Tuscany still awaits.

Printed in Great Britain
by Amazon.co.uk, Ltd.,
Marston Gate.